An Interpersonal Approach to Mental Functioning:
Assessment and Treatment

Contributions to Human Development

Vol. 20

Series Editor
Deanna Kuhn, New York, N.Y.

KARGER

Basel · München · Paris · London · New York · New Delhi · Bangkok · Singapore · Tokyo · Sydney

An Interpersonal Approach to Mental Functioning: Assessment and Treatment

Elsa Schmid-Kitsikis
Faculté de Psychologie et des Sciences de l'Education, Université de Genève, Suisse

English translation by *Hermine Sinclair,* Genève

1 figure, 1990

KARGER

Basel · München · Paris · London · New York · New Delhi · Bangkok · Singapore · Tokyo · Sydney

Contributions to Human Development

Printed in Switzerland by Thür AG Offsetdruck, Pratteln
ISBN 3-8055-5114-2

Contents

Preface

For a psychologist mainly interested in cognitive development, reading Schmid-Kitsikis's monograph is like suddenly discovering an altogether novel view of a building one had so far seen from only one perspective. I imagine that a converse shift of perspective will be experienced by clinical psychologists who read the monograph.

No psychologist, of whatever theoretical tendency, would disavow the links between emotional and cognitive aspects of mental functioning. But usually emotional experience is considered to provide the energy for cognitive functioning and development, rather than to shape and direct it. In Schmid-Kitsikis's view, affect also has a structural influence on cognitive processes. Notably, her work shows that symbolic representations of different kinds of experiences impose certain types of organization on the ways individuals construct knowledge. The importance she attaches to deeply rooted emotional symbols for the development of rational thought is both theoretically motivated and effectively demonstrated by analyses of her subjects' responses to a number of Piagetian tasks. The tasks are described in detail in Appendix A, some adapted to clinical practice.

In Piaget's own work, one finds certain references to subjective or egocentric thinking that ascribes to external reality the subject's (usually the young child's) own desires, fears and intentions, but one gets the impression that such subjective or 'autistic' thought is gradually eliminated during development in favor of 'communicable' or 'objective' thinking. In his very early work on language and thought of the child [1923/1959], Piaget contrasts the autistic and objective modes of thought [pp. 44–45] 'whose characteristics diverge so profoundly'. Taking the example of thinking about water, Piaget says that to objective intelligence, water is a natural substance whose behavior is subject to certain laws that can be studied, and that can be used in practical ways. To autistic thought, water is only interesting in relation to organic satisfaction (it can be drunk) and identified with liquids that issue from the human body.

> Thus in the one case thought adapts to water as part of the external world, in the other, thought uses the idea of water ... in order to assimilate it to more or less conscious images connected with fecundation and the idea of birth [p. 44].

When reading Schmid-Kitsikis's work, I was reminded of this passage, and looking for it, I came upon Piaget's footnote [p. 43]:

> There is interaction between these two modes of thought. Autism undoubtedly calls into being and enriches many inventions which are subsequently clarified and demonstrated by intelligence.

Piaget himself did not pursue this idea, but its far-reaching implications are brought to the fore in Schmid-Kitsikis's work in many illuminating ways. Indeed, affect and cognition interact, for better or for worse, and the complex processes at work, which Schmid-Kitsikis analyzes in this monograph, are realities that concern clinical and cognitive psychologists alike.

Genève *Hermine Sinclair*

Reference

Piaget, J. (1923): *Le langage et la pensée chez l'enfant.* Neuchâtel: Delachaux & Niestlé; translated into English (1959) by M. & R. Gabain as: *The language and thought of the child.* London: Routledge & Kegan Paul.

Introduction

In writing this volume, I was guided by two closely related intentions: (a) to give an account of my present theoretical reflections, and (b) to set forth my methods of psychological investigation and clinical practice. Theoretically, I aim to provide an analysis of mental functioning that combines the emotional and cognitive aspects of the subject's experience; in particular, I try to clarify the development and modes of functioning of creativity. In both respects, my practice as a clinical psychologist has proved enlightening.

The reader may wonder how the study of various deficiencies, inhibitions, deviations, etc., can help clarify the processes involved in creativity. Most studies of individual creative activities are based on an analysis of the finished product, rather than on the process that made the creation of something new possible. When creative activities are studied mainly as behavior leading to results valued by the social milieu, it is understandably difficult to grasp the subject's mental processes in their entirety. Once the truly constructive phase has begun, the subject is unlikely to exhibit the mental activity that is typical of the early stages of the process, with all its hesitations, trials and errors, inhibitions, and deviations. Instead of studying the finished products of creativity, i.e., original artistic or scientific works, which are always exceptional, my purpose is to explore the creative capacities of all human beings who discover and continually rediscover as yet unused (or only partially used) forces in the course of their development. These forces constitute the dynamics that drive the individual to develop mental activities whose absence leads to a state of inertia that annihilates developmental potential and can lead to 'mental death'. Clearly, genetic epistemology and psychology, with their emphasis on the study of the mechanisms of progress (in science in general, as well as in the development of the individual), contribute to the study of creativity in this sense, both through their research methods and their theoretical postulates. But what is the position of clinical psychology within this general framework?

Clinical Psychology and Piagetian Theory

What exactly is clinical psychology? Is it a method or an object of study? When the term 'clinical' was imported into psychology from medicine, ambiguities were introduced, and problems concerning the borders between psychiatry, psychopathology, and clinical psychology arose. According to Fedida [1968]:

> The fundamental problem of clinical psychology is less that of its relation to the clinical method in medicine than that of the foundations and the specificity of its various acts of perception, comprehension, interpretation and expression (p. 916, translated from original).

I am in agreement with Fedida's statement. When I started to use Piaget's work in studies of individual behavior, I became convinced that there was no reason to introduce into psychology the clinical attitude of the physician, but rather a need to reformulate the concepts and methods of psychology (particularly of genetic psychology), in accord with the needs that arise when the psychologist observes and tries to understand a particular individual.

In Piagetian investigation, the aim is to come to understand a subject's (usually a child's) development in relational and interactional situations that are as close as possible to experiences common to all. In clinical work, this approach is complemented by a search for the particularities of each subject's psychological and mental functioning, whether well-adapted, marginal or deviant.

Clinical psychology thus should not be characterized by its methods alone. The object of its studies and various applications has to be taken into account. In each particular case, the clinical psychologist relates what is individual to what is general and refers to discoveries made in other disciplines (such as developmental and differential psychology and psychiatry), in order to go beyond a descriptive analysis and to construct explanatory hypotheses.

From Genetic Epistemology and Psychology to Clinical Practice

My interest in the multifaceted processes and modes of mental functioning started from my acquaintance with the work of Piaget and his collaborators. I had the privilege of participating in various research projects concerning the development of knowledge, working with different age groups and in diverse areas of cognitive content. Later, my activities as a practicing psychologist, child psychotherapist and psychoanalyst of adults provided me with an additional source for theoretical reflection. Methodological questions, clinical observations and interpretations, and the discovery of certain phenomena led me further in the direction of an integrated theory of mental functioning, as I became increasingly aware of the close connections between affect and cognition.

This volume draws mainly on clinical work with subjects who encounter difficulties in the course of their development, an area in which the heuristic fertility of a constant interaction between clinical and theoretical reflection is particularly clear. Different aspects of clinical psychology – its theoretical approach, the collection of observational data and their interpretation – are treated in detail. All the chapters are concerned with certain conceptualizations that have guided my practical work as well as my theoretical reflection and that may be briefly sketched as follows.

Cognitive Difficulties and Psychopathology

In my clinical work with children, I noted an interesting convergence between observations made by teachers and those made by the psychologist during investigation and intervention. Indeed, the majority of children who present problems with respect to mental autonomization encounter difficulties in school. Their symbiotic, autistic modes of functioning or their exaggerated narcissism are accompanied by learning disabilities. Such children are able neither to create stable internal reference systems, nor to organize the external world confronting them. The fluctuations and oscillations manifest in their reasoning in Piagetian conservation tasks (involving the construction of invariants) invade all of their mental activity. A careful analysis of their mental processes reveals perturbations of the relation between fundamental mechanisms of development, i.e., assimilation and accommodation, and their links with libidinal drives. A study of cathexes and countercathexes and of the mechanism of splitting allows the clinical psychologist to distinguish various levels of cathexis which lead to 'hypertrophies', either of parts of the object, or of substitutive activity (choice of objects that have increasingly fewer relations with the original object), or of the treatment of the object (hyperassimilation and/or hyperaccommodation). The necessary links that allow the consolidation and integration of interiorized elements (fantasy, symbols, mental images, concepts) and that are necessary for well-adapted mental functioning cannot be established, and the subject's capacity for reflective abstraction, which leads to the mastery of one's own destiny as a thinker, is endangered, as well as the subject's symbolic activity and its creative possibilities.

The Role of Representations

The importance of mental representations and their development became particularly clear in my clinical work. Representations derive from various systems of psychic functioning (Freud's first topic), and for mental activity to be creative, representations should maintain links with their referents, i.e., early corporal, sensory, physical, and normative experiences. Corporal and sensory experiences reach back to the very first satisfactions of vital needs. From these experiences stem the first meanings created by the infant, giving rise to archaic representations sustained by the energy provided by affect. These meanings and representations are from the very beginning closely linked to the assimilation mechanism. They may, however, threaten to invade the total mental space. The subject then becomes unable to maintain contact with the external world without continuous interruptions by fantasy. The power of the archaic representations may lead the subject to hypertrophy assimilation at the cost of accommodation, and thus, simultaneously, to deny external reality and establish marginal meanings (characteristic of psychotic functioning), obstructing relations and communication with others.

Physical experience refers to experience with one's own or with others' bodies, with inanimate objects, and with the environment in general. The representations to which physical experiences give rise lead to the exploration and identification of objects. Analogous to corporal and sensory representations, they have to retain their links with material reality, so as to avoid an excess of reflective activity. Such excess can lead to an absence of exploration and identification of objects, in favor of their immediate classification, seriation, etc. At the other extreme, a low level of reflective activity can inhibit free association, anticipation and the creation of autonomous projects. Mental activity is then essentially accommodatory, and lacks distancing from external reality.

Normative experience refers to logico-mathematical experience. When the representations that derive from this experience maintain links with those derived from personal, sexual and cultural experience, they make the creation of powerful forms of organization possible. When rational thought does not maintain its links with affect, it becomes instrumental rather than creative.

The Integration of Experience

Only the psychic integration of these different kinds of experience and the representations that derive from them can render cognitive activity dynamic, open to new possibilities, and capable of novel creations. The theoretical perspective from which this claim derives is elaborated in the following chapters of this volume. The volume also provides clinical discussion, as well as an appendix containing detailed description of the various tasks used in my practice. I hope that the volume will serve both as an instrument for practical work and as a stimulus for theoretical reflection.

1

Theoretical and Clinical Contexts

A number of recent theoretical publications in French based on clinical experience have emphasized the importance of analyzing mental activity with respect to its functioning. Though this theoretical orientation was common enough in studies bearing on psychotic patients or severe mental retardates, over the last ten years it has also been seen in the analysis of so-called borderline mental functioning and cases of psychosomatic illness. Notable progress in the study of mental functioning has been achieved by authors such as Marty [1976, 1980], Marty et al. [1963], de M'Uzan [1977], Fain [1974], Braunschweig and Fain [1975], Kreisler et al. [1984], and others in the field of psychosomatic illness. At the same time, the French translation of Bion's [1962/1979, 1963/1979, 1965/1982, 1967/1983] and Meltzer's [1972/1977, 1975/1980] work led psychoanalysts interested in problems of thinking to reexamine Freud's sublimation hypothesis and the relations between sublimation and the sex drive. These new directions led to new theoretical proposals concerning the mental functioning of individuals who have difficulties in their relations with reality or who are suffering from psychosomatic illnesses. More important still, it led to the formulation of new hypotheses concerning the origins of mental functioning.

In many respects, my own theoretical and critical work follows the same direction. Clinical experience with 'marginal' subjects contributes, in my opinion, to our understanding of the mental functioning of the 'average' subject. More specifically, an application of Piagetian theory and methodology to the observation and treatment of patients allows the clinician to become aware of certain conditions that are necessary for mental functioning, and insight into these conditions leads to new hypotheses about the emotional origins of thought.

Clinical Observations and the Problem of Sublimation

The difficulties encountered by subjects who come to us for consultation are in the following areas:

(1) Cathexis of mental activity as an integral part of life. Our subjects seem to use 'thought' as if it were a foreign body.

(2) (Re)vitalization of cognitive schemes that have already been constructed and coordinated. In our subjects, it appears that no integrated link has been established between emotional experience and logico-mathematical and physical experiences needed to construct schemes that are formed when the child explores the world of objects.

(3) Use of trial-and-error activities that facilitate regulations. Our subjects seem fixated at the level of primary circular reactions, as if exterior objects could not be cathected as objects-to-be-known. They indulge in a profusion of repetitive actions that appear to be compulsive due to co-excitation.

(4) Activation of schemes of anticipation, centration, decentration and retroaction. These all call for representations. Our subjects' representations seem to be overpowered by mechanisms such as repression, denial, splitting, etc.

Generally speaking, the difficulties encountered by our patients highlight certain prerequisites for successful mental functioning: (a) the establishment of a psychical *space* for thinking, and (b) the elaboration of the *activity* of thinking. They also indicate that the sublimation process needs to be considered not only with respect to its final products but also with respect to its dynamics.

Using Piagetian theory both in clinical work [Schmid-Kitsikis, 1969, 1985a] and in research [Schmid-Kitsikis, 1987], I became aware of sublimation as an activity to be placed within a dialectic movement between cathexes and countercathexes, an activity that is linked to object relations and to the dynamics of the ego. The dynamics may structure and animate, or inhibit and disarticulate, though through various phantasmic, magico-symbolic or conceptual elaborations. If sublimation is generally considered to be a product of desexualization, it still needs to draw upon the libidinal sources of psychic activity in order to develop its force and its variety of elaborations and expressions.

I therefore tried to elaborate a theory of psychological functioning and its development in which cognitive activity and especially sublimation is considered in relation to fantasies and unconscious motivation. From this point of view, the study of mental activity must take into account both the internal psychic conditions and the contribution from the external world that insure its creative role. Several types of analysis derive from the fact that as psychologists we study the internal world of subjects as well as their relations with the external world. These include an analysis of mental activity that takes into account both its diachronic and synchronic dimension, an analysis of object relations and of the subject's interaction with objects, and an analysis of the contents of thought as well as of the processes of thinking. In clinical practice we thus, through observations and analyses, try to infer the psychological mechanisms that are at work and the nature of the subject's representational systems, in short, the subject's mental dynamics.

Investigation of the functional aspects of the emotive-cognitive elaboration of sublimation (whether well-adapted or not) is carried out through systematic exploration of what we call 'mental functioning', a term that encompasses both emotional and cognitive aspects and that suggests the existence of a functional center within which different types and levels of representation are elaborated and articulated, due to drive-determined cathectic processes.

The terms 'thought' and 'mental' are often used in a rather loose way in the psychological literature. 'Thought', in its more limited sense, consists of conscious reflection aimed at obtaining knowledge. In its wider sense, it consists of two types: (a) *private,* or autistic, thought, which is dream-like and depends on desires, affective needs and repressed elements that reappear in symbolic form; and (b) *directed* thought, focused on adaptation, which can be shared with others and which aims at rational coherence. Both in its narrower and its wider sense, thought is mainly analyzed through its conscious productions (reasoning, judgment, concepts, images, memories, symbols, secondary fantasies) and rarely through its processes. Only when thought is compared to activity is the question of dynamic processes taken into account.

The term 'mental' is traditionally applied to functions of regulation, storage and elaboration in the cerebral cortex or to the process of awareness that has its origins in physiological reactions. Consequently, the term 'mental' generally refers to perceptual discrimination, associative evocations, problem-solving activities, etc., and excludes both sensorimotor functions and the affective functions that guide the subject's behavior.

In our clinical practice we integrate the broad sense of thought with that of mental activity, and take into account drive (the Id), emotional origins of experience (such as those that lead to the elaboration of memories), diachronic and synchronic dimensions, and the transition between the moment of awareness and what precedes it. In this way it is possible to include in 'mental functioning' different types of object relations, diachronic and synchronic processes, and cerebral and drive capacity, along with their representations and symbolizations, as well as the higher forms of cognitive activity, which Piaget [1977] described in his study of what he called reflective abstraction.

This definition of mental functioning converges in part with the theoretical position of Bion [1962, 1967], who emphasizes the links between the emotional origins of the desire to think and to know, and the object that lets itself be thought about and known. Knowledge in this sense encompasses knowledge of one's self. The subject develops due to exchanges between emotional experiences and the models the subject uses in trying to organize contact with the external or internal world. The subject's approaches to the activity of knowing derive from these exchanges. Indeed, a theory of mental development and creativity should link processes that stem from object relations and drives, providing access to archaic forms of thought dependent on unstable private symbolisms, with processes that lead to sublimation via the cathexis of objects that are valued socially.

Representation

From this point of view, representations play an important part in mental functioning since they are closely linked to the drive dimension which is the source of all activity of the psyche. Representation in general is related to drives, to the body, to relational experiences and to the subject's encounters with the external world.

The general tendencies that give rise to representational activities can be described at earlier ages than Piaget proposed. Two phases may be distinguished:

(1) The child feels the need for physical contact with the mother or caretaker. If she is absent, the excitation continues and the child experiences displeasure. With the progress of sensorimotor intelligence (the formation of schemes, their coordination, the construction of objects and of space and time, etc.), the infant progressively becomes capable of assimilating inanimate objects to the mother and derives from them the pleasure she cannot give. The child chooses certain objects that were already meaningful in primary representational hallucinations and of which the child acquired a certain knowledge through accommodation. These objects are defined by Winnicott [1971] as transitional objects. A process of differentiation between the mother and the substitute object is set in motion:

Actions on inanimate objects may give rise to feelings of pleasure analogous to that felt in interaction with the mother, even though the necessary accommodation process is very different.

(2) Subsequently, the child may once again desire the mother and once again feel displeasure if she is absent. Substitute objects may also be absent, or they may have become inadequate precisely because they are inanimate. But even if the sensorimotor activity that brings pleasure cannot be pursued, the corporal pleasure can be cathected as an anticipation. There then ensues an interiorized imitation of this muscular or corporal activity, which becomes possible via the differentiation process that is already in motion. A second differentiation process then begins: The latent desire is dissociated from its actualization through substitute objects. The latent content thus assimilates the overt content and the subject feels pleasure by interiorizing its procedures (i.e., by functioning symbolically). These activities define a new level of mental functioning.

A certain quantity of drive energy is thus mobilized in order to construct representations that have to maintain their links with affects and relational objects in order to become dynamic and interrelated. In this way, sublimation can proceed, develop new adjustments and fertile recreations, and deal with the conflictual characteristics of the object and of the ego, as well as with object loss. Sublimation thus fulfills its function, i.e., it serves to elaborate symbols as creative links. These symbols relate elements of the internal to elements of the external world; meanings derived from the organization of emotional experiences are linked to the meanings the subject confers on external objects when acting on them, applying general constructive schemes (uniting, separating, ordering, etc., prefiguring the later logico-mathematical operations in the Piagetian sense). Symbolic constructions thus reach back to the earliest affective-cognitive experiences, their progressive articulation and reciprocal integration organized within mother-child interactions.

Mental Activity and Its Origins

This theoretical position concerning the development and functioning of mental activity thus combines concepts of genetic epistemology and psychology, of Kleinian psychoanalysis, and, more particularly, post-Kleinian theories such as those of Bion. It postulates that the origins of mental activity are to be sought in emotional, logico-mathematical and physical experiences and in their relations. The articulation of these three kinds of experiences forms a fundamental matrix that assures the subject's progress toward knowledge in the broad sense and favors mobility.

From birth, the infant is subject to different emotional experiences, in relation to internal as well as external conditions. These conditions allow the subject to form private representations. The experience of an object perceived as too menacing or too gratifying can modify, to a certain degree, the representation of its physical properties and inhibit or hypertrophy the organization of the actions the subject carries out on it. Since the breast or its substitute has particular physical properties (form, texture, size, odor, etc.) which the infant discovers due to repeated experience, a sensory and later mental knowledge of these properties is built up, both as knowledge of the physical object in the Piagetian sense, and as the cathected object. The infant experiences the physical world psychically, which Green [1987] explains in the following terms:

> What is psychic can only be engendered by the psyche, i.e., that of the mother; in other words, thought can only be engendered by the thought of the mother-object [p. 135, translated from original].

Since the infant is born into a world providing different stimuli, it is inevitable that certain stimuli will cause displeasure through either excess or deprivation. The infant will try to avoid displeasure and look for means to conserve or to restore a feeling of well-being. Using basic mental activities (uniting, separating, discarding, ordering), the infant acquires a certain power over both the external and the internal world. The coordination of the three types of experiences described above leads to mental activity that is emotionally fertile and conceptually controlled. In this way, affects can be integrated into the different levels of cognition and their associated representations.

Maternal Functioning and Infant Experience

My clinical data show that the three types of experiences (emotional, logico-mathematical and physical) are closely linked to two conditions of maternal functioning, the capacity for reverie and the function of the maternal protective shield.

Green [1987] interprets Bion's conception clearly. Bion [1962] proposes that the newborn is shaped by the digestive model derived from experience of the breast. In Green's terms, the mother 'digests' the projections of the infant's mind (she 'reabsorbs' them due to her capacity for reverie) and she nourishes the child in a different manner, with a preassimilated product. The mother absorbs the child's 'vomit' and does what the child cannot yet do: she 'psychisizes' this product into 'psychic nourishment'.

The infant can thus use this psychic food and construct the internal object while conserving the primitive psychic breast. From this foundation, the infant can create the conditions necessary for thinking.

In the previously quoted passage, Green defines both the mother's reverie (she reabsorbs the projections of the infant's mind) and her protective shield function (she transforms material food into psychic food that the infant can assimilate). The mother thus fulfills two conditions necessary for the psychic development of the infant: receptivity and capacity for transformation. If one of these conditions is absent or if their relations are inadequate, the mental development of the child may be endangered. As emphasized by Green [1987], the links between mother and child will then be unable to function as a basis for the construction of relations between relations, in other words, for the construction of thought. This approach converges with Piaget's concept of operations of thought as deriving from coordinations of action patterns.

Assimilation

When the relational conditions are fulfilled, the infant's experiences can become meaningful, representable and representative. The infant introjects the maternal reveries, thus allowing the development of assimilation, while the mother develops her reverie in harmony with her system of protective shield, which helps the infant to accommodate its activities to the properties of the external world, including those of the maternal world. In other words, a regulating system composed of gratifications and frustrations is established. The twofold maternal function of reverie and protective shield is thus at the source of an analogous system in the infant, composed of constructive trial-and-error activities (anticipations, gains, losses, etc.). When the various relational situations present a certain continuity, they engender the important assimilation mechanism. Piaget's postulation of the existence of an early capacity for integration and his analysis of the differentiations and coordinations by which the infant's most primitive activities are transformed into higher operations, as well as Klein's theory of the psychic work brought about by libidinal drives of linking, are both based on integration and assimilation, which allow incorporation, introjection and transformation, i.e., psychic activities supported by cathexes and countercathexes within the dual relationship of mother and child. The mechanism responsible for psychic communication between mother and child is that of projective identification, as described by Bion [1962;1967]. This mechanism allows children to discover gradually that they constitute a center of mental functioning that can act and have an effect on the environment.

Despite certain preprogrammed capacities of the infant, objects, with their physical properties and the actions they elicit, cannot be immediately differentiated. Only certain activities and their effects are recognized because they have caused pleasure or displeasure within a relational context; these will be repeated and consolidated, for better or worse. Thus, assimilatory activity is dependent on cathectic processes, and subjects will divide the psychic energy involved in their relation to objects and to themselves in various ways, according to the history and value of their fundamental experiences.

Frustration and Gratification

The affective-cognitive experience of satisfaction entails a desire for its repetition, but the experience of frustration, loss and absence (when relational conditions are not fulfilled and when objects-of-knowledge cannot be apprehended with the cognitive means at the subject's disposal) creates an internal need to supply what is lacking and to search for adequate means to satisfy desires when the mother is no longer available to provide and to transform. Like the inanimate objects whose resistance to become known was described by Piaget [1975/1977], the mother will also inevitably present certain resistances (frustration or losses), though her resistance is of a different nature, since a material object is far poorer in eliciting emotional responses (which exist only via the projective activity of the infant). Maternal resistance, alternating with maternal gratification, are the source of the child's endeavor to fulfill deficits or overcome obstacles, which is necessary for psychological development. The child's search for adequate means leads, on the one hand, to fantasy and symbolism (primary as well as secondary) through the mechanisms of assimilation and accommodation to internal schemes; on the other hand, it leads to the elaboration of preconceptual and conceptual thinking through the same mechanisms used in the construction of the relationships between the internal and the external world. Two creative processes appear that insure the development of imagination and of conceptualization. Their articulation and integration allow the elaboration of the symbolic world, both private and public. The degree to which the individual is able to mobilize his or her libidinal energy for constructive purposes is evidenced by various creations, but the latter do not by themselves reveal the means by which the process of elevation necessary for development is assured. It is essential that the replacement remain no more than an approximation of the desired object or event (desire for satisfaction or for knowledge).

The compromise between 'frustration' and 'tolerance' must allow for the existence of relational and/or cognitive dissatisfaction, in other words, for the desire to pursue the ideal state of total agreement or completeness without conflict which the subject attempts to reach without ever succeeding totally. This pursuit, which 'detaches' the subject from his or her partially satisfactory realizations and incites him or her to search for more efficient ones, is only possible through a mechanism that we call 'individualizing abstraction' [Schmid-Kitsikis, 1987], whose origin and development are to be sought in the activity of repression and in the binding of instincts, of representation and affects, of representations themselves, and of operations of thought. This repression and binding are assured by erotic forces and prevail over destructive forces so that anarchical functioning is avoided [Schmid-Kitsikis, 1985a, b, c].

Individualizing Abstraction

Individualizing abstraction permits relational and cognitive autonomization and avoids autistic and instinctual functioning as it is experienced in the enclosure created by the power of projective identification. Individualizing abstraction as a mechanism at work in both psychic and mental development allows the acquisition of the ability to wait, necessary for mental and relational anticipation; it also allows movements of ambivalence to avoid the mutilating connections between assimilation and accommodation, introjection and projection (through splitting, negation, etc.). It insures the pursuit of the relational object and of the cognitive object (as well as of their relations), which continue to elude the subject. It further insures the evolution of narcissism supported by psychic and mental movements that take into account the demands of the internal world in their relation with those of the external world.

The mechanisms of individualizing abstraction, the fate of which belongs essentially to the ego, become involved in the conflicts that surround ego development. Though the ego takes part in the search for the synthesis implied in narcissism (wish for binding and for the psychic and mental unification of itself), it is nonetheless attracted by the wish for unification with the object (relational fusion, mental accord with the object-of-knowledge). The internal compromise allowed by identification provides the means to escape imprisonment inside itself or the object (both relational and cognitive). This compromise takes place partly through the various expressions of archaic, symbolic, and normative thought. Thus, the ego comes to organize the fantasies that structure and animate thought and to allow the preservation of its links with the conditions of 'objective' reality. And, above all, it makes possible the articulation between the two organizing activities that give access to symbolic thought and that, despite their private character, can be transmitted on both the relational and cognitive levels by means of representations whose supports are to be found in referents (functional and structural, psychic and mental invariants) of a phylogenetic and ontogenetic nature. Primal fantasies, oedipal structure, conditions of object relations, mechanisms necessary for the elaboration of the internal world, and the construction of the cognitive object and the physical and spatio-temporal universe are involved in this process.

Meltzer [1972, 1975] and psychoanalysts such as Bégoin-Guignard [1985a, 1985b, 1988], who follow his theoretical model, provide at present one of the most interesting accounts of mental development through an analysis of the object relations (whose importance I discussed in the context of maternal functioning) and psychic mechanisms (such as projective identification) that govern it. Their analysis enriches the concept of individualizing abstraction. Meltzer's developmental perspective derives from what he calls the development of dimensionality in the representation the subject constructs of the world. He distinguishes four periods, of which the first two present conditions of uni- or bidimensionality that do not allow the subject to construct, in thought, different objects or events. At this level, a kind of psychic internal space is still lacking, inside which fantasy, as a trial act, and thus as experimental thinking, could take place. This lack creates obstacles for memory, desire and planning, as well as for a sense of time other than circular. Consequently, there is as yet no introjection or introjective transformation of objects; in other words, permanence is not yet possible. Only with the introduction of a third dimension do self and object acquire orifices, i.e., sufficient depth and openings to inject or expel contents. At this point, tridimensional representation of objects and, by identification, of self becomes possible, since both now contain potential spaces. Time becomes directional, from the interior to the exterior, and the subject uses, in an omnipotential way, the mechanism of projective identification.

Projective and Introjective Identification

Bégoin-Guignard [1985a] provides an interesting clarification of the process of projective identification. In her view, this process allows the subject to 'penetrate' into the object and

> to take possession of it in a more or less violent manner, to project one's self into it and to discard in it a component of the self in order to avoid an intrapsychic conflict (divide and rule!) or, by contrast, to use it as a secure place for storing that which in the self or in the internal objects could be attacked or destroyed by aggressive drives (p. 177, translated from original).

This process (derived from projective identification) ushers in psychic life, especially unconscious fantasy, and the fundamental symbolic function with the beginnings of secondary processes and language.

According to Bégoin-Guignard [1985a], no psychological life can 'be born without the help of another psychic life'. It is necessary to use 'one's projective identification' to 'dream' the psychic existence of another being. For Bégoin-Guignard, projective identification thus represents a genuine 'psychic respiration' because it gives 'meaning to relations with the other and with one's self'. In my view, this means that access to this process places subjects in a dependent state where they cannot exist without another being as well as in a state where they can progressively become themselves. This primitive kernel of symbolic functioning leads to Meltzer's [1975] fourth dimension, providing access to differentiation inside the self and to a new type of identification, introjective identification. The subject is now able to engage in personal creations, to construct and to symbolize, without discarding the elements that were at the origin of his or her psyche.

There is, in my view, a certain analogy between the process described by Meltzer [1975] and what I have called individualizing abstraction. The subject, freed from relations elaborated in play or by pure assimilation, accedes to a secondary relation that secures the infinite constructions of conceptual thought as well as the capacity to think one's own thought.

Piaget's Theory and Clinical Studies

The hypotheses that guide my research, theorizing, and clinical work are derived from the systematic application of Piaget's work to the study of mental functioning within the framework of interpersonal relations. Paradoxically, my hypotheses were suggested by the limitations of Piaget's theory with regard to emotional factors. Piaget's [1967a; 1967b; 1975; 1977] theory focuses on a subject who develops, makes discoveries, invents, and creates knowledge, but only the type of knowledge that is acquired either with minimal intervention of the emotions or due to a liberation from the emotions. Thought is considered to be progressively more and more objective.

Our clinical studies of both marginal and normal subjects helped us to understand the conflicts that develop when the subject tries to escape from the power of emotion. When this power is overly strong, the subject remains submitted to the influence of (amongst others) the first object relation. The study of the conditions of adaptation, of disharmony or dysfunctioning, or of psychological supernormality, shows how the subject progresses toward knowledge in the broad sense (of one's self, of others, of objects, etc.). Piaget's theory contributes to this analysis since it centers on both the functioning and the mental organization of the subject. Biological premises, the systematic construction of logico-mathematical operations and way of explaining these constructions help the psychologist to propose hypotheses concerning the various means used by the subject to survive and to develop mental activity in interaction with others.

Nonetheless, there remains a theoretical obstacle. In Piaget's theory, the subject has the desire to know from the very beginning. This is a fundamental cathexis particularly as regards objective knowledge. This primitive desire does not seem to need construction, and its development seems to proceed without obstacle, without detour, and without failure. Little room is left in the studies of Piaget and his collaborators for thought that escapes rationality and that freely follows associative paths. The subject of the Piagetian interviews is followed by the experimenter, sometimes assisted, sometimes contradicted, but only rarely left to his or her own devices. Moreover, the interviews yield a momentary view of a subject at a certain point in development, able or unable to solve a particular problem. What a particular subject can achieve in other situations demanding other constructions can only be inferred from what other subjects, in other situations or at other points in their development, have achieved. Piaget's theory describes possible subjects, having optimal functioning, provided with egos capable of development in a predetermined direction, and defined by their cognitive structures.

Nonetheless, my work on the mental functioning and modes of organization in the individual from a relational perspective has derived considerable benefit from Piaget's constructivist developmental theory. Using various tasks invented by Piaget and his collaborators, we have developed a way of analyzing and exploring the acquisitions and psychological realizations of our subjects. Our first aim is to understand the individual as a particular person, to capture his or her behaviors and to try to understand their meaning. We then proceed to a representation of the individual, taking into account his or her personal history and present state, including intellectual, social and relational acquisitions, characteristics of relational and cognitive functioning, and abilities to mobilize relational and mental potentialities during the process of clinical intervention.

Certain conditions are necessary for such an approach to be successful. In the first place, the encounter between the psychologist and the individual who comes for consultation involves processes of transference analogous to those between child and parent, therapist and patient, or teacher and pupil. The encounter is never neutral; it mobilizes unconscious forces on both sides. Though child consultations could be dual, they are in fact triangular, including psychologist, parents, and child. Parents are present at the conscious level because of their request for consultation. They are present at an unconscious level in the projection the child makes of parental figures onto the psychologist.

In the second place, the psychologist establishes a more or less conscious plan concerning the investigation and what will follow (treatment possibilities, their probable outcome, etc.). This plan comprises a system of representations (which will facilitate the process of transference) concerning the intellectual and relational future of the subject. Psychological treatment is therefore always preceded by a diagnosis as well as by a set of hypotheses concerning the possible development of the subject and implies an analysis of the essential condition for development, mental mobility. Three fundamental expressions of mental mobility may be distinguished – horizontal, vertical and functional.

Mental Mobility

Horizontal mobility is the subject's ability to vary his or her productions in the same situation, in other words, the variety of strategies and of solutions that are proposed, whether adequate or not, as long as the proposals indicate a search for solutions, and thus a certain degree of cathexis and an inclination to solve the problem. The subject's capacity to use and create mediators for the transmission of information and solutions is also important.

Vertical mobility concerns movements and transformations in solution-seeking or representational behavior at hierarchically different levels of elaboration. It is important to note the subject's capacity to alternate between regressive movements, linked to more primitive elaborations, and progressive movements linked to higher-level modes of elaboration.

Functional mobility is the subject's ability to go from one mode of mental functioning to another. Three such modes can be distinguished – projective, logico-mathematical and empirical.

The projective mode is characterized by behavior that attributes to others qualities, sentiments, desires or ideas that the subject refuses (consciously or unconsciously) to recognize in him- or herself. This mode of functioning can contribute to the process of knowledge when it is accompanied by a capacity to return to and into one's self, but it can become an obstacle for mental mobility when projection becomes a systematic defense mechanism against the anxiety caused by introjection (of elements that are perceived as painful, dangerous, etc.), thereby denying the internal world.

The logico-mathematical, or rational, mode is characterized by argumentation, judgment, justification, etc., which indicate a certain capacity to monitor or displace affects that might hinder the search for objective knowledge. This mode contributes to the development of knowledge in the broad sense as long as the libidinal sphere is not mutilated by excessive distancing and devitalization of mental activity. Mental functioning needs to safeguard its affects as the source that gives life to its representations.

The empirical mode is characterized by trial-and-error activities bearing on the external world. Though such activities are necessary in order to grasp the properties of objects, they can also become an obstacle to psychological individuation, which requires a certain cognitive and relational distance. Too many oscillations and fluctuations in behavior can lead to discontinuity and point to difficulties in the integration of the object-to-be-known, of the problem to be solved, or of the event to be reconstituted.

Various elements can be distinguished in these three main modes – a permanent or momentary dominance of primary assimilatory processes, through fantasy and magico-symbolic behaviors, or a permanent or momentary dominance of primary accommodatory processes, through clinging and mimetic behavior.

In order to analyze the subject's capacity to move from one mode of expression to another, two aspects of mental functioning need to be taken into account, the temporal and the formal. The temporal aspect calls for both synchronic and diachronic analyses of the subject's behavior. Synchronically, we note the subject's capacities for planning, for carrying out plans and for retroactive control, and the particularities of his or her tentative approaches to the problem. Diachronically, we analyze movements of progression and regression and their functional meanings (constructive regulations, contradictory fluctuations, breakdowns, instances of excessive control, etc.).

The formal aspect concerns the different modes of cathexis used by the subject and, specifically, the relations between assimilation/accommodation and projection/introjection. From the point of view of a broad definition of knowledge (of self, of others, of objects in the external world and of imaginary objects), two dynamic processes have to be analyzed and related to one another. On the one hand, the drive energy shows a certain direction and finality, and its mechanisms are those of projection and introjection. On the other hand, assimilation and accommodation are the mechanisms by which the contents of the internal and external world are transformed and which can lead to new knowledge. These transformations may be limited to a simple repetition of what exists already (e.g., circular reactions) or they can be the result of a change in the conditions for mental functioning.

The analysis of these mechanisms and of their relationships shows that their activity can lead, in a more or less stereotyped way, to the elaboration of three forms of abstraction, one of which may be privileged: (a) figurative abstractions (fantasies, imaginative symbols, mental images, etc.), which derive from the experience of satisfaction or dissatisfaction, due to lack or absence, and which open the way to the world of imagination; (b) logico-mathematical or normative abstractions (rules, laws, norms, consensual constructions, etc.), which derive from the experience of chaos and confusion (sensory, relational and mental) that leads the subject to organize actions and to become aware of the power to know the internal and external world; and (c) identificatory abstractions, derived from sensory and autoerotic experience (knowledge of specific properties of material objects, physical bodies, physical space, etc.), which open the way for exploratory and recognitive activities. Only when these three spheres of knowledge and their different abstractive processes are integrated can mental functioning become mobile and creative.

When the individual's modes and processes of knowledge are analyzed in this way, a better understanding is reached of his or her present functioning and potentialities for development. One can observe how the individual profits from learning situations, from the relational situation one can create, and from the cognitive stimulation provided by different tasks. These observations, interpreted within the theoretical framework sketched in this chapter, allow the construction of hypotheses about the quality of the subject's individuation and autonomization processes, as well as the extent of their completion.

2

The Psychological Meaning of Mental Constructions

In clinical psychology, a structural and dynamic analysis of the individual's basic mental constructions is essential. The psychologist needs not only to have access to the constructions the person with whom he or she is about to relate has already acquired, but also has to be able to understand the conditions that will favor this particular person's further development and nourish existing potentialities for individualizing abstraction. Such an analysis informs both diagnosis and prognosis, and facilitates psychological interpretation and intervention.

Several major difficulties pertaining to these mental constructions are frequently observed in our clinical practice.

(1) Certain notions and representations necessary for elaborating an internal world need to become permanent, in order to function as internal systems of reference, and this process of interiorization often encounters obstacles. When the mechanism of projection dominates introjection, the subject cannot develop the coordinations, integrations and differentiations necessary for psychological development. The internal world will remain chaotic, without stable reference points, leading to difficulties in memorization and in differentiation between sexes as well as between generations. Mental autonomization is endangered, as is the construction of an ego capable of development.

(2) The construction of the symbolic function, in its private as well as its conventional aspect, is impeded. The subject appears unable to create symbols that are based on links between representations and affects derived from emotional experiences, as well as from experiences with the external, physical world. Certain subjects can thus only reproduce representations that are commonly shared in his or her culture and that function in a consensual manner. Other subjects seem overwhelmed by phantasmic representations in which the assimilation process is dominant, and are almost incapable of establishing symbolic links with external reality. Such difficulties demonstrate not only the necessity of integration between emotional, physical and logico-mathematical experiences, but also the vulner-

ability of conceptual schemes vis-à-vis the powers of censorship and the economy of mental functioning.

(3) Mental images, through which the subject can reconstruct or evoke absent objects or events, are produced by the accommodation of assimilatory schemes in mental activity, according to Piaget's theory. In our subjects, the memory of such images appears to suffer either from excessive use of accommodation to the external characteristics of objects and events, which leaves no room for the necessary distance between reality and image, or from an excessive use of assimilation, which systematically distorts the links between image and reality.

(4) The development of conceptual activities is largely dependent on reflective abstraction. Here, again, our subjects encounter difficulties. They seem unable to activate the representations and the affects (as well as their relations) that are the fundamental components of conceptual schemes. Their thought thus appears devitalized, reified and disconnected.

In my view, these clinical observations support the theoretical postulate that it is necessary for an individual to use the life-giving source of the affects to construct meaning and to safeguard the links with cathected objects and their representations, as the basis for construction of a symbolic and conceptual universe, thus providing both a space and a creative mode for thinking.

Piaget's theory of cognitive development presupposes the existence of a mental space in which strategies are elaborated and decisions made in accordance with a memory base containing that which has already been acquired. Piaget himself [1970] refers to the 'cognitive unconscious'; this mental space (in the sense of a localization as well as a container) I prefer to call the 'preconscious,' where representations and actions necessary to mental development are elaborated. This space may be related to the two Freudian 'topics', of which the first (unconscious, preconscious and conscious) concerns intersystemic transformations and the second (id, ego, superego) the constitution of psychic instances. The two topics, particularly the ego and the preconscious, undergo transformations along different axes that can be compared to those Piaget defined to account for cognitive development. Piaget's theory postulates a first axis of coordinations, differentiations and equilibrations, and a second axis of reflecting and reflective abstraction [1975, 1977]. The first axis leads to the determination of different structural levels of equilibrium. The second provides access to reflection on one's own thinking. In this respect, in my view, there is a striking analogy between Piagetian and psychoanalytic theory (particularly that of Bion). Bion defined an alpha function responsible for links that transform primary and secondary processes, due to the work of the preconscious (coordinations, differentiations and equilibrations), for a container function assumed by the ego (the apparatus for thinking thoughts), which transforms the nature of its contents not only synchronically, but also diachronically, thus facilitating access to ever higher levels of what in our terms are called reflecting and reflective abstraction.

The Construction of Invariants

Many developmental psychologists interested in psychodynamics have insisted on the necessity of constructing invariants. But it was Piaget [1967] who demonstrated in the clearest way the importance of the mechanism of conservation, which leads to invariants whose permanence and continuity insure the individual's psychological progress towards increasing knowledge. By clarifying the conditions that allow a structure to 'continue to exist as a totality', Piaget showed at the same time how the subject can develop without feeling continuously threatened with dissolution, collapse or annihilation. Piaget considered the need for invariants to be particularly important in the domain of intelligence, since logical reasoning is based on the construction of invariant schemes used to organize the irreversible march of external events as well as the continuous flow of internal consciousness.

Other authors, such as Spitz [1965], Mahler [1973, 1980] and Winnicott [1971] emphasized the need for invariants in the area of object relations. They all refer to the processes that lead from an initial lack of differentiation toward a differentiated relationship via certain 'points of organization' [Spitz, 1965]. The processes are made possible by the internalization and stabilization of the mother (or her substitute) as a privileged object through the integration into one ambivalent object of what were earlier partial objects, experienced as either good or bad [Klein, 1932]. Later, these same processes lead to the final phase of psychological individuation, with intermediary stages of 'differentiation', 'habituation', and access to a 'differentiated object relation' [Mahler, 1975], stages that are reached through the creation of an internal object by the child, who is able to recreate an imaginary scene based on satisfying experience. Due to fundamental psychic experiences and the desire that leads to the imaginary recreation of these experiences, links are created between a certain relational reality as it is present in the history of the subject and the first manifestations of mental functioning.

This process needs to be linked to the 'intermediary area of experience', in order for the internal object to become stabilized without assuming a rigidity that would destroy its mobility. According to Winnicott [1971], these transitional phenomena are part of the realm of illusion that sustains the initiation into experience, and an important factor for change. The intermediary area of experience acquires a certain invariance when neither its link to external reality nor its link to internal reality are called into question. This invariance allows the ego (because of the prevalence of introjection and assimilation over accommodation) to remain uninjured by the conflicts that originate in the external world, just as in the cognitive sphere the invariants allow thought to be unaffected by threats of dissolution or regression and to grow both in extension and intension.

The initial dialectic movement between good and bad continues and combines with the differentiation of the sexes. The 'stranger anxiety' of the 8-month-old baby attests to a first differentiation of images of persons (as familiar or unfamiliar), but later the child will also realize that his or her relations with and reactions to father are different to those elicited by mother. This differentiation has to do with the internal objects that are linked to the oedipal organization. In the words of Perron [1985], 'the two parental figures have become sufficiently distinct to be related one to the other' and the child begins to feel the need to eliminate the parental figure that obstructs the exclusive love relationship with the other. This is the origin of 'the fundamental triangular figures of a three-person drama in which the union of two (child-mother, child-father, or father-mother) creates a dual relation based on the exclusion of the third' [Perron, 1985, pp. 71–72].

Representation of the self and of the object in its different forms (narcissistic imago, parental imagos, and images) is based on this development, which also leads to the construction of sexual, mental, and social identity. A kind of psychic space is created inside which play, representations, affects, thoughts, fantasies, dreams, and identifications can exist, through spatiotemporal processes necessary for the permanence of the self and the development of a psychological autonomy (individualizing abstraction). The development of identity is accompanied by the construction of invariants, diachronically as well as synchronically, and always in a dialectical manner.

The fundamental invariants are found in different areas of psychological development. The following can be distinguished:

(1) invariants that pertain to rhythmical activities and lead to the permanence of circular reactions, whether primary, secondary or tertiary [Piaget, 1936; 1937];

(2) invariants that pertain to objects independent of their movements and lead to (a) permanence of the relations between affects and representations of the maternal figure as observed in the phenomenon of stranger anxiety [Spitz, 1965], (b) spatio-temporal permanence of cathected inanimate objects, as observed in baby's recognition of objects when they appear in different locations [Piaget, 1937], and (c) permanence of the meaning of the representations attached to the so-called transitional objects [Winnicott, 1971];

(3) invariants that pertain to objects in movement, and that lead to (a) conservation of the cathected object when it disappears from the baby's visual field, as observed in search for the object [Piaget 1937], (b) conservation of the relations between the object, its displacements, and the subject's corporal behaviors that serve to reach it, as observed in the construction of the 'group of displacements' and its spatial structure [Piaget, 1937], and (c) conservation of the meaning of the links between representations established during the elaboration of what is called the transitional space [Winnicott, 1971];

(4) invariants pertaining to the object and its transformations, that lead to (a) conservation of certain properties of objects, such as quantity of matter, weight, and volume, that are left intact under physical transformations [Piaget, 1941], (b) conservation of relations between objects under logico-mathematical or normative transformations, leading to the concepts of number, classes and relations [Piaget, 1941; 1959], and (c) conservation of meanings of objects under transformations of substitution (in socioemotional situations), leading to the constitution of imagos, images and private as well as conventional symbols [Freud, 1900; Piaget, 1945; Winnicott, 1971]. Reversibility of thought and a stable differentiation between signifier and signified (in Piaget's terms) are made possible by this last group of invariants.

Our clinical investigations aim to determine the presence, the quality and the nature of three kinds of invariants: (a) socio-affective invariants; (b) the degree of autonomization reached in the course of individualizing abstraction; and (c) the relational and intellectual cathexes of the subject.

Various experimental situations can be used in these investigations. The well-known conservation tasks (Appendix A, A1–A8) elicit various interactions both on the relational and intellectual plane; associative play (Appendix A, B1) and drawing (Appendix A, A10) show the subject's projections and psychic and social representations. Other problems such as spatial problems (Appendix A, A9, C1, D8) and, in general, situations that require planning (Appendix A, D5, D7) can provide additional information. But conservation tasks, imaginative play and drawing are best suited to the investigation of the subject's identity in its relational, spatio-temporal, symbolic, social and rational dimensions.

Conservation Tasks

As used in clinical practice, conservation tasks allow the psychologist to assess the conceptual achievement of subjects and their use of a particular type of argument, but they also further understanding of subjects' mental identity when they elaborate and specify their thoughts during the interview. Several aspects can be investigated: (a) the nature of the relationship that develops between the subject and the psychologist during the dialogue; (b) the conflicts felt by the subject who is asked to think about a problem; (c) the conflicts that arise from the conceptual problems themselves; (d) the capacity of the subject to deal with conflicts; and (e) the status of the subject's acquisitions in the conceptual area under investigation compared to acquisitions in other conceptual areas.

Results obtained in one conservation task can only be interpreted confidently if certain behaviors are found to be frequent both in a single task and across different ones. For example, if the subject appears to be insensitive to counterarguments, it is necessary to ascertain whether such insensitivity occurs repeatedly but only in one task, or in several similar tasks, or more generally in other situations as well. The relational and interactive aspects of such investigations are sufficiently varied to allow the psychologist to discern functional particularities. The traditional Piagetian procedures are sufficiently intrusive and controlled to yield a clear idea of the subject's level of attainment with respect to the particular concepts of conservation.

The experimental procedures take the following course:

(1) Psychologist and subject agree on the equality of two sets of objects or of two objects as regards a particular property (numerical quantity, weight, volume, etc.).

(2) One of the sets or one of the objects is transformed (either by the psychologist or the subject).

(3) The psychologist asks questions about the relation between the transformed and the unchanged object(s). Is one more or less, or are they the same?

(4) The subject responds, either with silence, or with verbal answers, manipulations of the object(s), evasions, judgments, or arguments (either defensive or constructive).

(5) The psychologist asks new questions as a function of the subject's responses to earlier questions, and the subject responds again.

(6) The psychologist challenges the subject by proffering counterarguments.

(7) The psychologist continues the dialogue in order to evaluate the effect of the counterarguments on the subject.

The experimental procedure relies heavily on a question-answer dialogue (though some nonverbal versions, relying on gestural conventions, have been established by Furth [1964, 1971], and versions in which the subject is asked to act by Inhelder et al. [1972]). Though the predominantly verbal character of the tasks may be considered to limit, to a certain degree, their clinical usefulness, they remain excellent instruments for exploring both the conceptual achievements and the organization of the behavior of psychologically troubled subjects.

Reasoning

Two particularities of our subjects' reasoning are frequently encountered. The first concerns their preoccupations with the type of transformation the objects have undergone (pouring liquid from one glass to another, changing the shape of a ball of modelling clay, immersing metal cylinders in a glass of water, dissolving a sugar cube in hot water, etc). The second concerns their reactions to the use of particular objects (their degree of familiarity, of resemblance to real objects, whether they are animate or inanimate, etc.).

Transformations of Objects. The transformation of the object may be seen by the subject as its destruction or as an irreversible modification. When the ball of modelling clay is shaped into a sausage, it is impossible to return to the ball, because 'clay goes into the skin' or because 'the ball is destroyed'. When the sausage is made thinner and thinner, it will have 'no weight at all'. If a metal cylinder is immersed in a glass of water, the water level will not rise, because 'the water got stuck under the cylinder'. Similarly, a narrow glass can 'keep the liquid stuck', and a wider glass 'does not hold the liquid; it falls apart and you can no longer see it'. As the sugar lump is dissolving it disappears because 'there are grains of sugar that swallow other grains because they are stronger'.

These primitive answers seem to indicate that our subjects represent the events in conservation tasks as if they concerned the very existence of the objects. By contrast, when the objects themselves are not 'threatened', as in classification or seriation tasks, these same subjects are sometimes capable of operatory reasoning.

Representations of Objects. Some of the objects traditionally used in the conservation tasks (lemonade, chips, modelling clay, etc.) seem in our subjects to produce representations that block the investigation. The subjects attribute meanings to the objects that are either too threatening (snakes, bugs, etc.) or too disagreeable (urine, feces, etc.). At other times, they seem incapable of accepting a non-realistic representation (a little wooden cow becomes a real cow who eats real grass; chips are exclusively for playing a game, etc.). Interestingly, changing the objects (tiny beads instead of lemonade, candies instead of chips, etc.) is sometimes sufficient to enable the subject to accept the situation as fictive ('as if') and to respond to the psychologist's questions.

It thus appears that subjects whose psychological functioning is troubled, and, though less so, subjects who have learning difficulties at the cognitive level, face a basic problem, that of cathexis (of the objects, of the conceptual field, of certain types of thinking, etc.). Thought cannot function generically as long as it remains dominated by particular objects, events and environmental conditions. Individualizing abstraction cannot take place.

A word of caution should be added. The psychologist should not hastily conclude that a subject is incapable of reasoning along certain lines, since a change in the objects presented can change the subject's behavior. At the same time, the subject's particularities should not be minimized, since they provide insight into the state of elaboration of the self.

Organization of Behavior

An analysis of the ways subjects organize their approaches to the task indicates two main difficulties, stabilization of their arguments (whether they are adequate or not) and use of stable systems of reference.

Oscillation in Argumentation. Throughout one task, with its sequence of questions, answers, suggestions, etc., subjects will continue to question their own main arguments by proposing contradictory statements. The main argument can be one that affirms conservation ('There is still just as much clay'), or that denies it ('No, this one has less'). At the same time, subjects give answers that contradict this main judgment. These oscillations are not comparable to those of normal subjects who are at a stage of transition. Our subjects produce such contradictory patterns of response in several conservation tasks at different levels of cognitive achievement. They behave as if they suffered from an inability to make a decision, because they are afraid of failure and of assuming responsibility for following a certain line of thought. Or they seem to suffer from a lack of continuity, as if they apprehended their world in segmented portions, introducing the notion of many equivalent possibilities and rendering contradictory judgments equally truthful.

Fluctuation in Argumentation. Fluctuation is different from oscillation as defined above, in that it does not pertain to subjects' argumentation about one particular item in the task, but rather their reasoning about different items presented during the interview. Subjects change their judgments from one situation to another, so that, for example, the same container can be said to contain first more, then less, and then the same amount of liquid as another, or a first transformation can be judged to change the amount, a second not to change it, etc. Once again, this fluctuation does not indicate that the subject is at a transitional stage, since it appears in different conservation tasks, as well as in those that pertain to the construction of invariants at a simple level. There appears to be a general difficulty of maintaining one response, whatever the status of that response.

Instability of Systems of Reference. To compare numerical quantities or physical properties, one needs a system of reference. In conservation tasks, a transformed object is compared to an untransformed object, which serves as a reference point, as do certain measuring instruments (e.g., the scales used in the conservation of weight). These objects and their properties have to be thought of as stable, and our subjects seem to have difficulties in recognizing this stability. For example, in the task bearing on the dissociation between weight and volume, they seem to 'forget' that the psychologist changed the cylinder that was immersed in the water, but that nothing was changed as regards the water; they may say, 'The water goes up higher here, because we put in more water'. In other tasks, these subjects constantly change the object that serves as a reference point for comparison. Again, such instabilities are observed in our subjects in conservation tasks of different conceptual levels.

The difficulties encountered by our subjects appear to fall into two categories: (1) in relation to the objects used in the tasks, and (2) in relation to the organization of thought. In the first case, the subject's relation to the objects is dominated by the emergence of archaic fantasies (incorporation, morselling, etc.). A surfeit of assimilation gives rise to an extensive system of representations. Objects are felt to be threatened or threatening, and the lack of differentiation or distance between subject and object results in the subject feeling threatening or threatened. The subject's thinking thus appears saturated with corporal and magical elements.

In the second case, the lack of continuity in the subject's thinking, as evidenced by the oscillation, fluctuation, and instability of reference systems, appears to be due to the dominance of the mechanism of splitting over that of linking. The subject appears to avoid the stabilization of a system that establishes links both between the subject and the object and between elements of thought, as if, paradoxically, this stabilization were felt to be a dangerous subservience to the object.

Investigation of Mental and Sexual Identity through Analysis of Drawings and Play

Private and social representations are best captured in interview situations, in imaginative play, or in drawings, i.e., in situations in which the subject can give free rein to associative processes. Since representations are cathexes (issued from memories of early experiences), they are related to memory systems. Private representations are related to primary and secondary narcissism, to the degree of internalization of the self, to the ideal self, etc. Sociocultural representations, derived from the system of identifications, combine that which pertains to the oedipal structure and the influence of the environment.

The conservation tasks already provide certain insight into the subject's representational and conceptual systems, as has been shown, but other situations are necessary to clarify the state of the subject's imagos, images and identifications, as well as the nature of the link between subject and object (phantasmic, symbolic, etc.).

Associations Produced during Play

One of the situations used in our clinical practice is that of play (Appendix A, B1). The same situation has been used in a study of normal children's symbolic development [Schmid-Kitsikis et al., 1987], oriented towards exploring the construction of symbols. The study allows an analysis of the prerequisites necessary for symbolization, i.e., the construction of an internal world made possible by the permanence of certain acquisitions. In this respect, it provides insight into the quality and nature of the psychological identity of the subject. Methodological details regarding analysis of the observed behaviors can be found in the paper by Schmid-Kitsikis et al. [1987]; here, those observations that are significant with respect to clinical practice will be described.

The following collection of miniature objects is used: (1) toy people (man, woman, baby), (2) toy animals, wild (crocodile, bear, dolphin) and domestic (wolfhound, rabbit), some made of hard plastic (crocodile, dog), others of furry material (rabbit, dolphin, bear), (3) food and kitchen utensils (bread, carrot, baby bottle with milk, knife, spoon, mug, pot with lid), (4) toilet (WC) and toiletries (comb, mirror), (5) tools (spanner, pincers, scissors), (6) doghouse, and (7) objects that have no socially defined use (an open cube made of plastic, modelling clay, a piece of cloth). The subject is encouraged to play with these objects as he or she likes. Only if the subject focuses on actions such as sorting, grouping, separating, etc., does the psychologist suggest, 'Can you play a story?'

In general, the psychological difficulties of those who come for consultation are related to the fact that they attribute personal meanings to the objects. The properties certain objects have in the external world may be dominated by the personal representations they elicit in our subjects, who all, to a greater or lesser degree, present a fragility of the self. All of them have difficulties in differentiating the external from the internal world, and in controlling primary processes so that they neither intrude on secondary mental activities nor become too isolated. According to the degree to which drive energy is linked to representation, the latter can become either too archaic or too conventional.

The play session may provide information concerning the differentiation between the subject (either as an observer of his or her imaginative play or as a participant) and the story being staged. In short, free associative play provides material for analysis of (a) the links between fantasy and play themes, (b) the prevalence of certain mechanisms (projection-splitting; assimilation-accommodation), and (c) especially, the nature and quality of object relations, of the degree of integrity, and of the narcissistic autonomy of the subject.

Example: Olivier's Play at Age 7. In the following description of a play session, a certain number of details are left out to permit a focus on activities that are important for our analyses.

(1) Olivier explores the material. He picks up, one after the other, the dog, the dolphin, the woman, the man, the toilet and puts them down again. He then takes the doghouse, puts the dog inside it, puts the loaf of bread inside the pot and the rabbit inside the plastic cube, adding the carrot.

(2) Olivier stages a happening in the family. He spreads out the white cloth and sets down the man and the woman next to one another; then he has them lie down. He puts the modelling clay underneath the man's head as if it were a pillow. He then puts the baby next to the doghouse and adds the baby bottle. He then lays the baby down next to the man. He takes the cloth and covers baby, man, and woman. He tries to take the shoes off of the woman and of the man. He puts the bear next to the baby.

(3) Olivier acts on the baby. He takes the baby, opens the toilet and tries to put the baby inside, using force. He then takes the baby bottle and tries, violently, to put it into the baby's mouth. He stops, looks at the milk in the bottle, and puts the bottle back into the baby's mouth while looking at the bottle.

(4) Olivier acts on the dog and the baby. He takes the doghouse and tries to get the dog out of it, using pincers. He succeeds, then takes dog and baby and has them walk side by side. Then he places the baby on the dog and has the dog jump. He puts the dog back into the doghouse, tries to get the baby in as well, fails to do so, and puts the baby under the cloth.

(5) Olivier acts on the woman and the man. He tries to take off the man's shirt. He looks at his feet. He folds the legs of the man and of the woman and puts them side by side in a kneeling position. He puts the man and woman back upright. He brings the hands of the man in contact with those of the woman. Then he lies them back on the ground. He lifts up the man, lifts up the legs of the woman, touches the neck of the man and the genital area of the man, and brings the leg of the woman down. He turns the woman and the man around, and then takes the carrot and puts it in the rabbit's mouth.

He takes the man and the woman again and places them facing and leaning one towards the other. Then he has the man fall down, and the woman move on top of the man. He says, 'He is dead'. He mimes a fight, then lays the man down again, puts the woman on top of the man, and then puts both back upright.

He lays the man and the woman on the cloth and the baby between them. Then he takes the woman and lays her down at the edge of the table, so that her head hangs over the edge. He lays the man down on top of her, then next to her. He rolls up the sleeves of the woman, opens her legs and stretches one of her legs in front. He lifts up the woman and the man and places them upright, the woman with her foot on the genital area of the man. While doing so, he grimaces and blows air from his mouth. He mimes a fight.

(6) Olivier announces that he will straighten out the messy house. He rearranges the objects, including the animals and people.

(7) Olivier acts again on the man and the woman. He lays down the man and the woman and announces that they are going to do 'silly things'. He once again mimes a fight.

A detailed analysis of the protocols of two other children is given by Schmid-Kitsikis [1985, pp. 139–151]. In this paper I will only discuss those behaviors that can provide insight into the psychological constructions of Olivier's internal world.

From the beginning, Olivier acts as an observer and stage manager. In this role he explores the objects and stages several happenings (family scenes, fights, etc.) with great realism. His status as a subject who is the center of mental functioning is clear, and the relations and coordinations necessary for the dramatic performance are present.

His themes belong on the one hand to daily life (food, clothing, sleep) and on the other to his fantasy life (all-powerful maternal imago; aggressive mother able to kill the father; narcissistic imago sometimes deficient and crushed by maternal violence – the baby is forcibly fed, thrown into the toilet, and incapable of stopping fight between the parents though placed between them). Although Olivier sometimes obeys his repetitive fantasies (the primitive fight scene appears to be the central theme of his play), he is also capable of resisting and readopting his position as an observer. The differentiation between the internal and the external world is relatively well-established, even if at times the projection and the accommodation to his subjective fantasies may dominate. Similarly, the differentiation between the sexes is established, though the representations are inverted, since the mother possesses the greater physical power. What seems disquieting is the content of his projections, indicating that his identification with the paternal imago is not propitious to his development as a little boy.

Associative Productions in Drawing

Compared to the play situation, drawing has the advantage of calling on the subject's internal world without the need for objects other than the drawing material, but it is difficult to interpret below a certain level of technical proficiency, especially when unaccompanied by comments.

Various techniques are in common use. The subject may be asked to make a drawing on a particular theme (e.g., 'draw a family') or may be left free to choose a theme. I discuss here drawings that resulted when subjects were asked to draw a sequence of six episodes, depicting what happens to a child during a day when the child is free to do as he or she likes (Appendix A, A 10). The protagonist of the story will no doubt present certain projected aspects of the subject, thus permitting the psychologist to evaluate the permanence of the psychic identity of the subject, through an analysis of the procedures used, the affects and judgments, the relational and social behaviors, and the internal reference points of the identificatory movements.

Example: Drawings by Gilles at Age 10. Gilles drew eight episodes instead of six (fig. 1). When he had finished he commented on his story.

Gilles draws well; his narrative is clear and follows the drawings. He has an extended vocabulary and uses sophisticated expressions to formulate the relations between his drawings and the intentions of the characters. An analysis of such drawings needs to take the following aspects into account: (a) the representation of time and space; (b) the expression of affects; (c) relational and social elements; and (d) identification movements. As for the play situation, not all details will be given in this paper; an extensive analysis is given by Schmid-Kitsikis [1985, pp. 151–156].

With respect to Gilles' drawings, the following points can be made:

(1) Time and space are represented with precision. The sequence of events and their different locations follow the plot correctly. A woman is out for revenge, she pursues Gilles, and carries out her criminal intent while taking precautions not to be suspected. Caius is aggressed, abandoned by his mother, cared for in an institution and then killed by the vengeful woman. The events are sequentially localized: Caius coming out of the house, the road, the hospital and finally the cave.

(2) The theme of the drawings is treacherous vengeance by a woman who makes sure that she will not be suspected. It is also a story of loneliness and of someone unable to defend himself.

(3) The affects expressed are the following: for the woman, pleasure in revenge, hate, treacherousness, and power; for Caius, innocence, loneliness, suffering, and impotence.

(4) Several relational and social elements are clearly expressed. Caius is abandoned by his mother, who leaves him in the hands of strangers. She does not come to the hospital with him and prefers to go and look after her burning cookies. A curious crowd gathers and disperses when there is nothing further to be seen. Caius is shown suffering in bed all alone, surrounded by machinery that identifies the institution.

(5) The identification movements (identity and identification with parental imagos and images) express the differences between generations (there are adults and the child, Caius) and between the sexes (there are the women, Caius' mother and the mother of his classmate, and there is the child, Caius). In the drawings, however, these differences do not appear; all the characters are represented as stick figures. Gilles seems to have focused on the story rather than on figurative aspects of his drawings. The maternal imago and image occupy the foreground. Although socially the mother is represented as a good housewife who bakes cookies, Gilles' maternal imago is powerful, frightening, hateful and cold-blooded, synthesizing his own mother and the mother of his classmate.

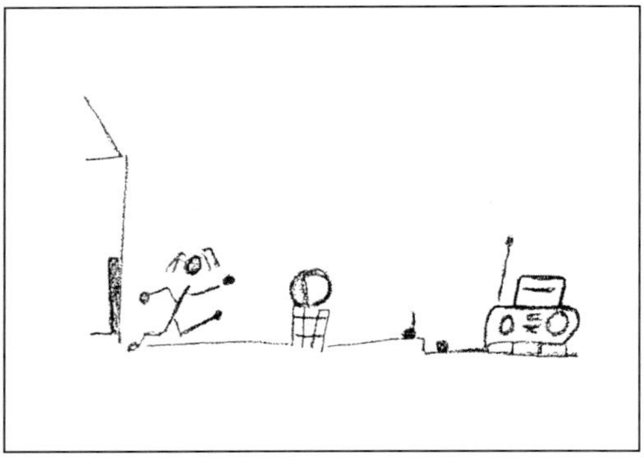

Fig. 1/1. A boy called Caius comes out of his house. A woman, the mother of one of his classmates, who has been expelled from school because of Caius, has decided to take revenge on Caius. During the night she placed a nail at the edge of the sidewalk in front of Caius's house, to make him fall. She is on the lookout for Caius, sitting in her car.

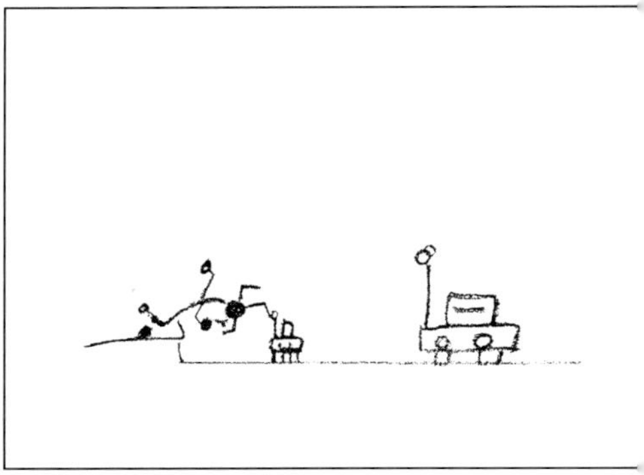

Fig. 1/2. Just as the woman expected, Cai stumbles over the nail and falls. She starts drivi closer to him.

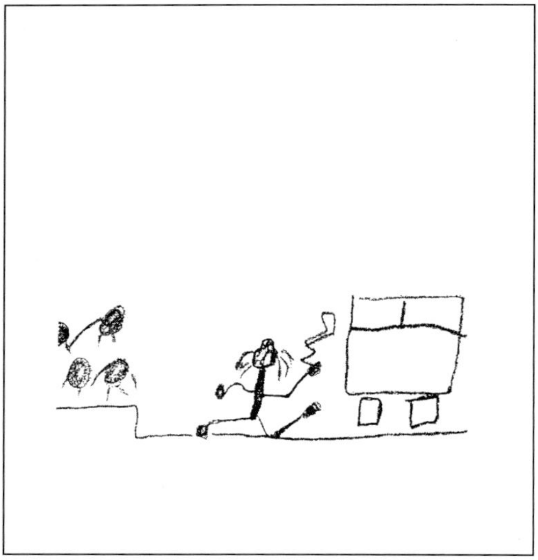

Fig. 1/5. The ambulance leaves with Caius. His mother remains at the side of the road. The crowd disperses.

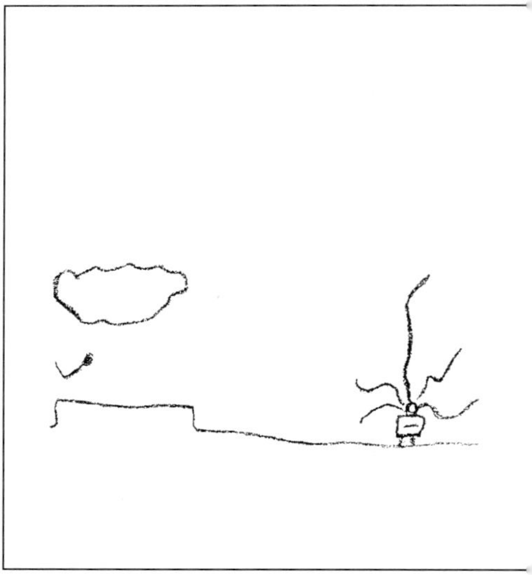

Fig. 1/6. Caius's mother goes back into t house, because she sees smoke. The cookies a burning. The ambulance disappears in the di tance.

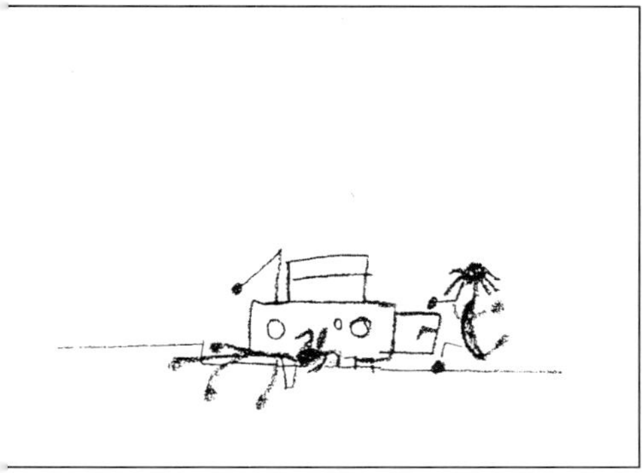

Fig. 1/3. She accelerates and drives into Caius ho is lying in the road. Caius is seriously wounded. ne antenna of the car is broken. The woman gets t of the car and pretends to be surprised at the cident.

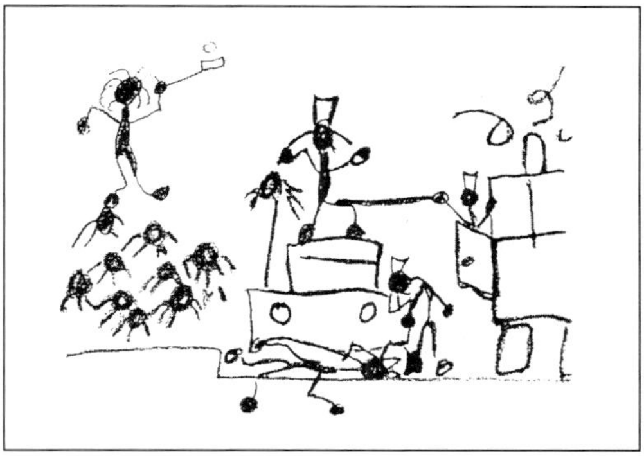

Fig. 1/4. A crowd gathers around Caius. Somebody calls for an ambulance. Caius' mother, alerted by the noise, comes out of her house, a pan in which she was preparing cookies in her hand. The ambulance arrives. The woman who caused the accident pretends to faint. She remains close to the ambulance in order to find out where Caius will be taken.

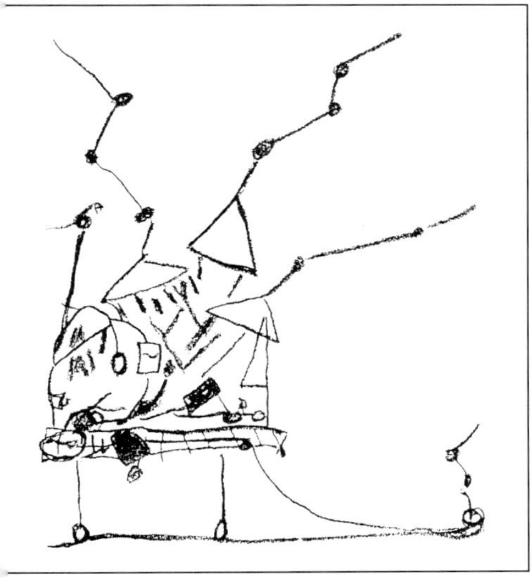

Fig. 1/7. Caius lies in his bed in the hospital surunded by many apparatuses – surveillance camas, an intravenous drip and a respirator. He is riously ill.

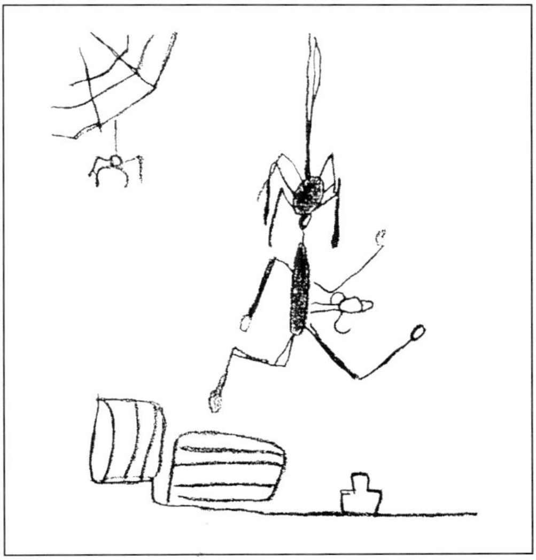

Fig. 1/8. During the night, the woman comes to the hospital and kidnaps Caius in order to go and kill him in a cave. She strangles him, hangs him, and sticks a sword into his abdomen.

In summary, the three tools that have been described, conservation tasks, free play, and drawing, allow us to observe essential characteristics of mental functioning in different spheres of psychic life, with respect to the reference systems and the stability of subjects' physical, spatio-temporal world, their relational and social, as well as conceptual, representations, and their identificatory systems and movements.

The Symbolic Function: Its Construction and Psychological Meaning

Analysis of the fundamental invariants of development illuminates the progressive elaboration of a psychological identity, which becomes organized through the unification and consolidation of the representation of objects and of the subject's own self, as well as through the construction of conceptual schemes. The analysis of symbolic elaborations provides an introduction to the creation of meaning by way of the various expressions of necessarily ambiguous contents. Though interpreting symbolic productions remains difficult because of their ambiguity, this difficulty stimulates the search for substitute constructions, which the subject elaborates according to his or her relational and cognitive experiences, and leads to the characterization of the subject as a 'user', 'reinventor', or 'creator' of symbols.

In Freud's [1900] theory the elaboration of symbols is considered a creation of the psyche, and it is evidence for various compromises, constructed so as to make it possible for antagonistic psychic processes to function together despite their differences.

Construction of Symbols

Analysis of the construction of symbols pertaining to the construction both of the ego and of the object has been carried out mainly by the developmental psychoanalysts, such as Spitz [1965], Klein [1930], and Winnicott [1971]. If symbols are indeed a creation of the ego, allowing a metamorphosis of the anxieties engendered by object loss, then this creation cannot be immediate but must depend on relational development. According to these authors, the main phases of this creation depend on certain significant experiences:

(1) Experiences that engender in the baby the thought 'I am the breast' via the care received from the mother figure as a container and a protective

screen. This experience allows the baby to focus on his or her own body, or the orifices and the skin, through ex-corporation and in-corporation.

(2) Experiences that cause frustration or a feeling of loss and that force the baby to search for an object that brings satisfaction. The desired missing object (the breast) has to be recreated by the baby. The experience of lack or loss thus leads to symbolization. The recreative activity is the source of symbolization, but it is not in itself a symbolic representation, since for the baby to fantasize the breast is equivalent to possessing the breast. Baby and mother are still fused, and consequently signifier and signified are not yet differentiated. In Segal's [1957] terms there is a 'symbolic equation' at this level.

(3) Experiences that elicit symbolic representations issued from the dislocations that gradually separate what is fantasized from what is perceived in reality, between the function of the mother as a container and those of the mother as a libidinal figure. These differentiations lead to a growing awareness of the relative inadequacy of fantasies versus reality. Such dislocations, or ruptures, in the relational continuity are necessary for self-integration, though, paradoxically, the mother has to remain mentally available to the baby in order to heal the traumatic loss and to make the baby feel that the link with the mother is unbroken.

(4) Experiences that help the baby to distinguish between being linked to an object by way of projection and using a real object perceived as different from the self. These experiences lead to fantasies in which the object is destroyed but resists its destruction, thereby creating the conditions that make it possible for the baby to use the object as something different from the self and thus to symbolize it. This symbol for something different from the self can then be used for communication.

(5) Experiences (as described particularly by Winnicott, [1971]) that, with the help of maternal reverie and reverie of the environment, lead to the construction of a potential space, an intermediate sphere of individual experience, which becomes the kingdom of illusion and creative play and of cultural and artistic activity.

Access to symbolization therefore announces object permanence. The baby who imagines the object's destruction and then is able to recreate it attains a certain stability of privileged representations, such as those of the maternal figure. But this progress entails internal conflicts (anxiety, ambivalence), because the mother can be felt both as good and as bad – as the mother who nourishes, rocks and calms, who gives meaning to the baby's body, emotions, and gestures, and as the mother who frustrates and abandons the baby. The baby's dependence on the mother creates ambivalence in relation to the instinctual drives. The experience of the alternation of presence and absence, of pleasure and displeasure, engenders the anxiety of loss and the struggle for the recreation of the object through introjection and assimilation (keeping the mother inside oneself in order to restore her). The recreation of the object leads to its symbolization and the displacement of aggression onto an object other than the mother herself, at the same time protecting her against the child's aggression. The distance thus created between self and object makes it possible for the baby to be alone in the mother's presence as well as with her in her absence.

For Piaget [1945, 1966], the symbolic (or semiotic) function consists of the capacity to evoke something absent (object, person, event) by means of a signifier (word, gesture, image) that is differentiated from its signified. This capacity also allows the representation of currently absent, but formerly experienced, properties of present objects or events. Piaget distinguishes motivated symbols (which conserve a certain link to what they represent, such as certain gestures or drawings) from arbitrary symbols, such as words, numbers, formulas, graphs, etc. Piaget described five different kinds of behavior, of varying degrees of complexity, that indicate the advent of differentiated signifiers: (a) delayed imitation, (b) symbolic (or pretend) play, (c) drawings, (d) mental images, and (e) language. Two of these, imitation and symbolic play, illustrate the relations between accommodation and assimilation particularly well. Imitation uses and prolongs the accommodation to various phenomena and objects perceived in the external world.

In Piaget and Inhelder's [1966] theory, mental images originate from overt imitation, in the form of signifiers-in-action. Progressively, imitation can be delayed and take place well after the object or event has disappeared. This detachment from the here and now leads to the construction of a variety of mental images, or actions, and thus to the beginnings of representation. Even when the representation is an action carried out in the here and now, it can be used to evoke the absent phenomenon. For Piaget, the beginnings of representation belong to a level that is intermediate between evocative actions and genuine mental representation. Mental images, as copies or internal reproductions of objects or events, are the product of interiorized imitation.

Symbolic play is, in Piaget's theory, a construction that complements that of imitation. In individual symbolic play, children construct meanings guided mainly by the process of assimilation. Symbolic construction in play proceeds in a parallel way to the construction of mental images through imitation. Since in symbolic play the child develops the feeling that he or she acts 'as if', free from the constraints of the external world, this pretense can be used as a means of satisfying cognitive and affective needs that cannot be fulfilled when the child is trying to adapt to reality.

A more detailed review of psychoanalytic and Piagetian conceptions of symbolization as the construction of a system of meanings is presented by Schmid-Kitsikis [1985a]. The present discussion is limited to the important question that emerges from comparison of the two conceptions. Are all creations of meaning symbolic, so that meaning and symbolism are interchangeable terms, or is there a difference between them? More particularly, does the capacity for symbolization develop under specific conditions not necessary for the construction of meaning in general?

According to Klein [1930] and Winnicott [1971], symbolization is a dynamic psychic activity with an integrative function, which takes place in a particular mental space, different from the space that allows the construction of copy images, or fantasies, that are the direct expression of a conflict between drives and their meanings. This point of view leads to an analysis of differences between symbols with respect to: (a) the distance between signifier and signified (e.g., in their temporal relation or with respect to level of meaning); (b) the nature of the substitution or of the mode of access to the signifier (e.g., a simple copy image vs. a transformation based on analogy); and (c) the extension of the relational links (e.g., a one-to-one correspondence versus a correspondence via a third element).

Symbolic Functioning

An analysis of symbolic behavior that takes into account the above-mentioned points contributes to our understanding of the organization of the subject's psychological functioning. In my view, two essentially different modes of functioning can be distinguished in various situations that elicit symbolic behavior, such as pretend play or drawings – that of the subject as *user* of symbols and that of the subject as a *reinventor* or *creator* of symbols.

Symbol Users

Certain subjects seem to limit themselves to an excessively accurate reproduction of reality and of the conventional ways in which their community experiences it, as if established rules should never be broken and nothing can be expressed except what has already been 'learned'. They seem to have constructed an identity imposed from outside, as they are seen by others. They seem to deny the existence of an internal world and its possibilities for individual creations, and to make excessive use of accommodatory mechanisms and of 'absorbing' meanings that are organized and adopted by the collectivity. From the external world they accept only such elements as already have a conventional value or are apt to fill a gap left open by a deficiency of linking.

In my view, this type of functioning – the inability of the subject to elaborate 'genuine' symbols – can be interpreted in two ways. On the one hand, it may be supposed with Gibeault [1982] that part of the ego is identified with the object, through the projection mechanism, and consequently, the symbol (or what should be a symbol) is identified with what it symbolizes. The substitute object is thus experienced as if it were the original object, and it is no longer possible to recognize and to accept that the substitute has its own properties, different from those of the original. This converges with what Segal [1957] calls the symbolic equation.

On the other hand, according to a different but related hypothesis, part of the ego is identified with physical and normative characteristics of the object, also through projection. In this case, the symbol, or what should be the symbol, is identified with its formal or 'dressed up' appearance and no longer exhibits its dynamic, personal features. The subject consequently experiences sociocultural and normative forms as if they were his or her own creations.

In both cases the identity of the subject and his or her capacities for symbolization are endangered, either by an excess of assimilation (since the symbolic object given by the environment is experienced like the original internal object), so that the reality of the subject cannot be insured, or by an excess of accommodation (since the symbolic object created by the subject is experienced as if it possessed the properties of the external object), so that the reality of the object is too dominant. These types of functioning can indicate the subject's entry into a psychotic or pre-psychotic stage, through dissociations or the installation of a false self. The future of the subject's capacities for symbolization, and, consequently, for individualizing abstraction, is thus at risk.

Reinventors and/or Creators of Symbols

By contrast, subjects in the second category rediscover, in the course of their own development and their encounters with often unforeseen situations, the symbolic elaborations that are indispensable for communicating with and relating to the external world. The reinventor of symbols constructs what others constructed earlier, and what others will construct in the future. The developmental conditions for this type of functioning have been described by Piaget [1945], Bates [1979] and Winnicott [1971], according to whom reinventors of symbols are, to a certain degree, the agents of their own development. They elaborate internal and external processes of differentiation that condition the emergence and the evolution of their symbolic activity, while remaining in close contact with the models provided by the environment and their own interpretation of these models within a system of interaction and communication. They thus create an internal world that also contains conventional representations, insuring links with the environment.

One of the conditions for the creation of such an internal world lies in the acquisitions made through activities of imitation and delayed imitation, which create meanings that favor the construction of self and other. Imitation and delayed imitation joined to other mental activities become dynamic processes, indicating that the subject is capable of elaborating symbolic representations based on the links he or she establishes with conventional internal and external models, opening the way to new creations.

By contrast, the imitative behavior of subjects that are only users of symbols seems to lack such an opening towards further development. Indeed, the users of symbols constantly reveal their dependence on products of imitative activity, which may be due either to hypercathexis of this activity (with limitation of its fields of operation) in order to assimilate and reproduce idealized adult behavior, or to the absence (through disavowal) of the transformation work underlying the assimilatory activity (felt to be too conflictual) and the dominance of the accommodatory activity of imitation, delayed in time.

I wish to emphasize the developmental aspect of the two types of functioning that have been portrayed. It may be that from birth (and even before birth, via the parents) the baby lives in a certain environment with its specific cultural, social and biological characteristics, and this environment uniquely determines the child's future as a user of accepted symbols. Or, there may exist environmental conditions that lead the baby towards a future as reinventor or creator of symbols.

The user of symbols has failed to construct his or her 'being' as a center where cathexes and countercathexes needed for the individualizing process are related. The reinventor of symbols, in contrast, reconstructs the phylogenetic and cultural heritage and becomes an individual with ego autonomy who fits into the environment in which he or she lives. This achievement opens the way to a new role, that of creator of symbols, who can combine originality and tradition, seeking what is already known and established by others as well as what is different and original.

Development of this creative type of functioning depends on two conditions: (a) the psychic integration of the subject as a member of a traditional community with a collective past and as a particular individual with a personal past; and (b) the inescapable link between creative symbolization and mourning. Kleinian and post-Kleinian psychoanalysts, such as Klein [1940, 1952], Winnicott [1935], Meltzer [1972, 1978], and Segal [1981] have emphasized the relation between the development of symbolism and mourning. In their view, creativity rests on the activities that aim at reconstituting object and ego – on the desire to recreate lost objects and to reconstruct what has been destroyed. These processes favor the development of relations and constitute the basis of thought. In a certain sense, this idea of the existence of lack or absence as important for the development of symbolization is also found in Piaget's theory. Having reported several as-if behaviors in one of his children, Piaget [1945] asks a question:

> Why would she imitate the movements of a church bell, or lie down stiffly like the dead duck she saw in the kitchen, or try to make her doll – a recalcitrant baby – eat pretend soup? The answer is clear: The child's thinking is not yet sufficiently precise and mobile, her logico-verbal thinking is too short-lived and vague, whereas the symbols make everything concrete and lively (p. 162, translated from original).

Both in Kleinian and Piagetian theory the creation of symbols is thus considered to arise from a real or potential experience of absence or loss. On the one hand, this experience is real since it follows the actual experience of the 'good' object and of primary satisfaction. On the other hand, it is only potential because it depends on the absence of what is not yet present – later logical thought, whose absence leaves the subject in a mental state of chaos. In the first case, there is psychic suffering, an essential loss that calls for the work of mourning; in the second case, there is mental chaos and anarchy, calling for a search for equilibrium.

Creators of symbols are therefore dependent on representations derived from their own personal experiences, as well as on representations provided by the persons who directly participate in their development (parents or their substitutes) and by their sociocultural milieu. In this way, they are able to enter into relations and to communicate with others. Creators of symbols appreciate the complex alliance between different memories – that of the subject's own experience, that of the environment in which he or she lives, and that of the species which underwrites his or her origins.

Mental Images: Their Elaboration, Function and Psychological Meaning

In the discussion of symbolization, I referred to two aspects of mental images. On the one hand, mental images play a part in the acquisition of knowledge, and on the other they function as memory devices for what has been perceived in the external world (and/or in the actions of the subject), serving the subject's desire to restore what was before and what is now in the near or distant past. For Piaget, images help to communicate to others what is perceived, but their main function is to serve various adaptations through recapitulation. Mental images are also cognitive behaviors whose development can be followed. They provide a means of studying cognitive development through understanding of the relations between image and knowledge.

Theoretical Perspectives

Prior to the beginning of the 20th century, psychologists considered thought to consist of associations of images. Only with the advent of experimental methods did a new view of thought come to the fore. Psychologists began to realize the complexity of thought and recognized the existence of thought without images. Mental imagery seemed less interesting, partly because experimentation in that area proved difficult, and psychologists began studying logical thinking. Meyerson [1932] reinaugurated the study of mental images as symbolic instruments of thought, but it was not until 1964 that a paper appeared in English, entitled 'Imagery: the return of the ostracized' [Holt, 1964]. During this time, Piaget was carrying out research on the development of mental images [1964] and on long- and short-term memory [1968]. Piaget is one of the few authors during this period to have proposed a comprehensive theory of mental imagery; many others carried out research in this field, but without, in my opinion, offering a comprehensive theory [Cooper & Shepard, 1973; Dick, 1974; Horowitz, 1970; Hoffmann et al., 1973; Neisser, 1972; Paivio, 1969, 1977; Richardson, 1969; Segal, 1971, 1972; Sheehan, 1966, 1972; Steiner, 1983].

Piaget, however, studied mental imagery only from the point of view of its links to cognitive development. Few authors [Euse and Haney, 1975; Huckabee, 1974; Singer, 1966] have tried to treat mental imagery in its relation to the emotional sphere. When mental images are studied in relation to cognitive memory, the subject's cognitive structures that have become permanent, and thus remain available for representation, have to be taken into account. Working from this point of view, Piaget and his collaborators [1966] came to the conclusion that mental imagery is subsequent to perception and that it follows different laws: it is a *reconstruction.* Of course, mental images are not directly observable; various means are used, such as drawing (which despite technical difficulties may provide the most trustworthy access), gestural reproductions (which can often clarify drawings), and verbal explanations (which sometimes indicate better-adapted images than can be inferred from drawings, though they may often remain rather vague, since the subject mainly expresses a global understanding of the perceived phenomenon). The research by Piaget and his collaborators led to a certain classification system. It appeared important at different degrees of complexity to distinguish images that derive from *static* objects or forms, those that bear on *displacements,* and those that bear on objects or forms that undergo *transformation* in the course of the experiment.

Two aspects of Piaget's theory of mental imagery are particularly important for clinical diagnosis: (1) the mental availability of what is acquired and the subject's process of selection; and (2) the substitution carried by the image. Mental imagery necessarily implies a reference to objects (or events) in the past or the present. Images have a function of reference, derived from the imitative activities that allow the subject to evoke, reconstruct or reconstitute a past or present object or event, as well as a function of elaboration [Denis, 1979] that creates new content or new relations with content that in the past experience of the subject gave rise to images. These new constructions can, in turn, acquire a referential function.

The conditions of the environment or of the personality of the subject can lead to a dominance of one of these functions over the other, since both functions are intimately linked. For some subjects, the referential function may be dominant, since they cannot allow themselves to construct novelties and only restore repetitively what was experienced in the past. For other subjects, the function of elaboration may become dominant; they rely on imagining a possible future, as if this behavior provided refuge, control, liberating distance, etc., from conflictual reality.

When the coordination between reference and elaboration becomes perturbed, resulting in the dominance of one over the other, an analysis of the processes of assimilation and accommodation can lead to a better understanding of the active role the subject adopts toward knowledge. Though images derive from imitation, and thus constitute an activity of accommodation, assimilation is always present, and their reciprocal relations are necessary for equilibration – the main process of mental structuring. According to this view, the study of mental imagery provides deeper insight into the coordination of assimilation and accommodation than the study of the subject's reasoning and rationalization. It allows an analysis of mental process, and an analysis of the subject's capacity to create a continuity between figural units that are perceived successively in a certain context and to introduce spatial and temporal discontinuities into events that are perceived in a continuous manner. It is far superior to a verbal interview in providing insight into the status the subject accords to reality and to his or her internal world.

The substitutive character of imagery explains why it is considered to be a specific component of representative structures and thus part of the symbolic function. Since in Piaget's theory images are studied in their relation to cognitive development, they are defined as evoking figural aspects of reality, which implies a certain schematization and approximation. Images, therefore, remain in the figurative sphere of cognitive activity, and play only a limited role in the construction of object knowledge. The more important operative aspect, i.e., the logico-mathematical understanding of transformations, provides the foundation on which symbolic representation can become an actual tool of thought.

The differentiation between signifier (image) and signified (object or event), if considered as a process rather than from the point of view of its products, remains a powerful factor in the transmission of meanings. These considerations led me to make a distinction between different kinds of images as symbolic representations. On the one hand, there are symbolic representations that serve the *recognition* or *identification* of objects or events in the immediate or distant past, which the subject wants to reconstitute as faithfully as possible; on the other hand, there are symbolic constructions that create new *relationships,* in line with those already established. In the first case, images are called upon because of their figurative fidelity, but they limit the user's role as an active observer of his or her own memory; in the second case, the more complex symbolic representations derive from *transformations* carried out on different memories – those of the subject's own past, the past of the environment and the past of the human species, i.e., the subject's biological and phylogenetic origins.

Semiotic ambiguity (but not figurative fidelity) allows such transformations to take place and protects the psychic and mental identity of the subject. This is an important function, but its impact on the construction of objective knowledge is far from obvious. For this reason, Piaget and his collaborators have focused on the type of semiotic instruments that serve the faithful transmission of reality.

The Study of Imagery in Clinical Practice

Since we have insisted from the first that the emotional sphere should be taken into account in the study of mental development, the question arises as to why we make use of Piagetian tasks, limited as they are to the sphere of objective knowledge. In the absence of a mental imagery theory based on experimental evidence that could link mental images to affects and show the influence affects have on memory productions, we use Piagetian tasks (Appendix A, C1 to C3) in two ways, that allow us to determine: (a) the *quality of the subject's mental disposition* in the face of the psychologist's request; and (b) the *capacity* of the subject to *exploit* the experimental reality (the objects, instructions and spatio-temporal conditions presented) and to *remedy* its insufficiencies.

The experimental situations allow an analysis of the mental disposition of the subject in so far as his or her activities are related to: (a) the interplay between assimilation and accommodation; (b) the links between foresight and retroaction; (c) the differentiation between viewpoints; and (d) the segmentation of the movements or transformations of an object or event into imagined units. Mental images are most adequate when they account for manifestation of reality in the most objective way, and their construction depends on a mental state in which emotional activity is controlled. Though this mental state is partly determined by the subject's cognitive acquisitions, it also depends on the quality of the subject's encounter with the psychologist. Certain subjects are capable of reasoning in terms of their stabilized cognitive acquisitions, but not when the situation has to be explored beyond already interiorized logico-mathematical systems.

Several tasks demand such explorations of the particular experimental situation. The problem of the construction of mental images of the shadow produced by a rotating circle or slanting stick, for example, can only be solved through a close analysis of the particular experimental situation. This difficulty explains – at least in part – the lag between conceptual and imagined activity that is observed in subjects that are preoccupied or psychologically unstable.

The same experimental situations also allow analysis of the subject's capacity to exploit reality and to remedy its insufficiencies, through the study of: (a) the subject's handling of the proposed situation (e.g., asking for help, avoiding conflicts, using surrogates); and (b) the use of intermediaries such as material or instruments that are not provided in the task but are introduced on the subject's own initiative.

Such procedures reveal the difficulties the subject experiences, but also the power of activation of his or her ego. It is important to observe whether the subject is able to find ways and means to deal with the task situation or whether the subject is overwhelmed by the difficulties.

These are the only aspects of mental imagery that a Piagetian interview can reveal, since the experimental situations do not provide access to the images' power of elaboration (with one exception, to be discussed later). The nature of the tasks does not allow the creation of new relationships, but only a reproduction of objective reality; new constructions can only be distortions. Moreover, since the objects used in the experiments are neutral (geometric forms, beads, sticks, etc.), they elicit an appeal to cognitive functions without suggesting anything personal, except in the case of certain particular dysfunctions. The situations are thus equally new or equally familiar to all subjects. A constructive image is needed to anticipate the result of a transposition or transformation, but this still concerns the immediate future.

In my opinion, it is precisely the neutral, ahistorical character of the Piagetian tasks that allows us to understand two important aspects of mental disposition: (a) the semiotic constructions already acquired during development; and (b) how the subject functions at the time of the psychological investigation. Similarly, the neutral, ahistorical conditions allow the psychologist to observe either behaviors of compensation and supplementation or behavior indicating regression or even collapse. Such observations enrich understanding of the adaptative systems employed by the ego when faced with conflict.

In this way, clinical interviews with children and adults made us aware of the degree to which certain chronic or transitory psychological disturbances can handicap or disrupt mental activities, particularly those involved in solving spatial problems. Solution of problems requiring mental imagery appears to be especially disturbed in the case of depressive, psychotic, borderline cognitive and phobic states.

Logico-Mathematical Thinking: Its Construction and Psychological Meaning

Investigations of logico-mathematical (or normative) thinking have always been part of clinical interviews. Indeed, clinical psychologists agree that, whatever the social and cultural origins of subjects, their thinking must show a development toward the objectification of knowledge, toward a detachment from various subjective factors. Although intuitive and associative thoughts are supposed to be the sources of mental creativity, these modes of thought, if they dominate, usually are not regarded as adequate beyond a certain age.

Theoretical Perspectives

Piaget, more than most, emphasized the development of logico-mathematical thought. He showed that logical thought becomes more and more powerful, with the various integrations, differentiations and generalizations that develop via self-regulatory processes of reflective abstraction, and also that other fields of knowledge, e.g., space, time and causality, are organized based on the same logical structures and via the same processes.

Piaget was particularly interested in the relations between two types of knowledge, knowledge about the physical world and logico-mathematical knowledge. Both types of knowledge have their source in experience, but two aspects of experience are to be distinguished: (a) physical experience, during which the subject acts on objects and discovers their properties and relations (e.g., observing that pieces of wood float in water but pieces of metal do not), and (b) logico-mathematical experience, during which the subject draws knowledge not from the objects themselves, but from the way he or she organizes or transforms the objects (e.g., arranging objects in a row, counting them, then rearranging them into a square, counting again, and finding that the number remains the same).

Physical knowledge, even at the highest levels, always requires experience, but at the same time it is based on a logico-mathematical structure (if only to organize the investigation, to treat the data, and to construct laws), but logico-mathematical knowledge can become 'detached from the objects and function symbolically with purely deductive operations' [Piaget, 1967b, p. 385]. Logico-mathematical knowledge functions through reflective abstraction, whereas physical knowledge is based on 'simple' abstraction [Piaget, 1967b].

Though the construction of logico-mathematical knowledge remains for a long time dependent on experience, its roots go back to the beginning of life. During the first days after birth, the infant already 'distinguishes and recognizes among the many impressions he receives from his world certain stable groups which we will call "pictures"' [Piaget, 1937, p. 10, translated from original]. These perceived pictures (either visual, gustatory, tactile or auditory) succeed one another, and, especially, they disappear. In that case, there are two possibilities:

> either the picture is immediately forgotten, i.e., it disappears into affective nothingness, or its loss is regretted, it is desired, and the infant awaits its reapparance; the only means to make it reappear is to repeat the accommodations that were made before [Piaget, 1937, p. 17].

Moreover, these 'pictures' have as yet no depth or relief: they are only 'spots that appear, move and disappear without having any solidity or volume' [Piaget, 1936, p. 63]. Interestingly, this view of the first mental matrix is shared by recent authors who work in the psychoanalytic tradition and who use concepts such as 'primary mosaic' [Marty, 1980], 'psychic unidimensionality' [Meltzer, 1975] and 'beta elements' [Bion, 1962].

According to Piaget, the first cognitive activities of the infant consist of isolating from these syncretic pictures 'certain clusters of qualitative elements that are relatively stable thanks to repeatable actions (the beginning of action schemes) leading to the constitution of objects and relations' [Piaget, 1937, p. 195]. Further development during the sensorimotor period leads to the many achievements described and discussed by Piaget [1936, 1937], such as the gradual elaboration of object permanence, spatial structures, and physical causality. Important aspects of this development emphasized in these works include the 'function of implication' as present from the earliest activities of the infant and as the basis for the development of logic: 'All acts of intelligence suppose systems of mutual implication and of shared meaning' [Piaget, 1936, p. 14]. Much later, this idea was elaborated further by Piaget and Garcia [1987] and led to a new interpretation of Piaget's logic of operations as a logic of meanings, closer to a logic of relevance and necessity [Piaget and Garcia, p. 173] and less limited to traditional extensional or propositional logic.

From this perspective, the early phases constitute a proto-logic, during which 'the instruments of deduction in the proper sense are prepared as evidenced by the formation and coordination of the first assimilatory schemes, i.e., the first implications between meanings' [Piaget and Garcia, 1987, p. 14, translated from the original]. Subsequently,

> whenever the subject is confronted with a new situation, an interaction takes place during which the subject apprehends the empirical data provided by the situation through the use of the logical organizing instruments already constructed during earlier experiences. The use of these instruments renders the empirical data observable in the sense that they are interpreted and organized. Each new situation encountered and interpreted by the subject will in turn contribute to the construction of new instruments for assimilation, i.e., logical instruments, that will serve the interpretation of other situations [Piaget and Garcia, 1987, p. 154, translated from the original].

During development, there are thus periods of relative stability, when the subject becomes capable of dealing with unavoidable perturbations (internal contradictions, new problems), aided by already constructed logical instruments. When this is no longer possible, there will be disequilibration and

> reorganizations (reequilibration) that bring the system into new stationary conditions ... the system fluctuates ... under the influence of internal or external variations. Beyond a certain limit these fluctuations engender the system's instability ... (disequilibration) [Piaget and Garcia, 1987, p. 156].

This interpretation of the development of logical structures in terms of meaning structures retains assimilation as its most important mechanism, since it confers meaning both on objects and on actions. The meaning of objects can be defined as what one can *do* with them (i.e., to what action scheme or conceptual scheme they are assimilated); (b) what one can *say* about them (i.e., their description); and (c) what one *thinks* about them (i.e., their classification, relations to other objects, etc.). The meaning of actions is defined as what their result is according to the transformations they impose on objects and situations. The meaning of actions is thus linked to the subject's interaction either with external, physical realities or with entities constructed internally (such as logico-mathematical entities). The logical relations established by the subject are (either at the level of actions or at the level of propositions) based on *implications between meanings.* Theoretically, i.e., from the point of view of the observer, they are combinations of implications and negations. In other words, 'at all levels the foundations of logic are inferential, which is obvious in a logic of meanings' [Piaget and Garcia, 1987, p. 191].

As explained by Piaget and Garcia [1987, pp. 183–186], Piaget's logic of operations was never totally convergent with propositional logic; its convergence with entailment logic, or 'logic of meanings' is clearer. From the psychologist's point of view, a logic of meanings constitutes a most welcome elaboration of Piaget's idea of action schemes as meaning-giving elements and of his adoption of Claparède's concept of 'implication' (entailment) as the psychological activity that makes it possible for the subject to profit from experience [Piaget, 1936]. What is emphasized in the 1987 work by Piaget and Garcia is the view of the psychological subject as an individual searching for and interpreting meaning.

This search for meaning introduces the problem of the relations between affect and representation, since the relations arise from internal activity that links past acquisitions (i.e., cathected experiences that leave meaningful traces) to present acquisitions that thereby in turn become meaningful. The logical activity of the subject, i.e., the organization of experience, is thus carried out on experiences that have mobilized the subject's affects and led to certain representations.

Clinical Investigation of Conceptual Structures

The clinical investigation of conceptual structures informs the psychologist about the way the subject organizes his or her mental actions. Its object of research is the state of knowledge of the subject as a center of mental functioning and organization. The subject's actions, their coordination and elaboration, and the subject's awareness of his or her activity and capacities for development also inform us about the quality of his or her narcissistic universe and the movements of the libidinal forces of linking and unlinking.

Two aspects of such investigation are particularly important. The first is determination of the subject's conceptual acquisitions – of the underlying operations and their actualization. The second is analysis of the dynamic expression of the subject's interaction with the environment – his or her capacities for resolving conflicts and creating novelty. The first aspect informs us about the state of attainment of logico-mathematical structures and about the systems the subject has constructed and that have been mastered by his or her ego. These systems enable the subject to confront the resistance of reality and the ensuing conflicts. The second aspect helps us to understand the subject's conceptual procedures and the links between them and activities in other domains.

The analysis of behavior that is dynamic and constructive (in the sense of its being the result of the way the subject deals with conflicts) reveals the following types of functioning: (a) the search for equilibrium and objective coherence, in order to deal with conflicts, leading either to resolution and new constructs, or, at the other extreme, to denial; (b) the search for an approach to the problem through reflecting or reflective abstraction, in order to facilitate the narcissistic process, and leading either to elevation or, at the extreme, mutilating isolation; and (c) the search for efficacy and permanence, through anticipations and retroactive verifications of the planning process or, at the other extreme, refusal to make decisions.

The most important type of functioning for the development of mental activity is that of reflective abstraction. This process leads the subject to mental constructions that are increasingly independent of particular behaviors in particular circumstances, that are increasingly turned towards the subject's own thinking as an object of reflection, and that thus contribute in an important manner to development of the ego. Analysis of this type of functioning is clearly related to that of the development of the ego image in the narcissistic sphere.

Though there are different forms of reflection or reflective abstraction at different levels of development (with a shift from focus on content to focus on form), reflective abstraction is present at all levels. The subject gradually discovers him – or herself as a thinking person, who has constructed certain types of thought and who can create new contents and forms of thought on the basis of what is already acquired.

For analysis of the subject's logical thought we used Apostel's [1959] categories: classifying, relating, judging, and inferring. The generalizing power of these behaviors can indicate the existence of a search for coherence, with 'truth' as its main objective. Absence, or deficiency, of these behaviors in situations in which they are elicited can indicate the dominance of libidinal forces whose discharge or intrusion is irresistible.

The Psychological Meaning of Classification, Construction of Relations, Judgment, and Inference

(1) Classification activities have important psychological meaning, particularly when they are observed in spontaneous behavior or, at least, in situations in which classification is not explicitly suggested. They reveal the desire of the subject to master the situation by using various components of classification. This is done by generalizing, identifying and organizing the different properties of material objects, and by adopting an economical procedure that avoids useless losses or gains. In tasks in which classification is requested by the psychologist, such activities are much

more difficult to observe, since the problem is imposed from the outside. Classifying behaviors are analyzed by tasks D2 to D4 (Appendix A).

(2) Construction of relations is part of most mental activities and hence more difficult to grasp through particular tasks (Appendix A, D1, D8, D9). In general, the activities of subjects in these tasks inform us about the way subjects use and organize internal and/or external figurative models and acquire concepts and their components. This analysis accounts for the quality and the nature of trial-and-error procedure and linking processes that are guided by a plan or project and that thus demand anticipations, verifications and modifications, as well as use of information provided by the material elements of the task.

(3) Judgments are difficult to observe in other than verbal forms. They generally involve the initial searching and transforming activities of the subject before a decisive response can be produced. They inform us about the subject's capacity to perform mental actions *before* and *during* the organization of the problem's elements that is necessary for its resolution. Though the subject has to form judgments in all tasks, only certain tasks instruct the subject explicitly to do so. Conservation tasks are of this type. Analysis of the subject's behavior focuses on the judgments and supporting arguments produced during a series of transformations carried out by the psychologist or subject.

(4) Inferences are part of the deductive or inductive reasoning process that leads to the construction of norms. Inductive reasoning implies an integration of what is carried out in the present (or the near past) with the future. Tasks (Appendix A, D5, D6) involving inductive reasoning provide occasion for the subject to anticipate, to plan, and to verify. They allow the psychologist to observe the points of view the subject adopts provisionally (hypotheses) and the procedures adopted to elaborate them further and to verify them. In addition, they assess the subject's capacity to construct a reasoning process that links propositions adopted at earlier points in the task to the final judgment.

In these tasks the subject has to maintain a constant mental alertness, since the psychologist hardly intervenes. The solution of the problem lies in the more or less distant future, and the subject has to pass through a sequence of intermediate discoveries that are to be related to one another. This necessity can be a source of anxiety, and inefficacy or lack of mental alertness can result in constant interruptions, necessitating repeated verifications. Such behavior informs the psychologist about the ways the subject tries to integrate emotional with logical activity.

Dysfunctions of Logico-Mathematical Thought

The characteristics of logico-mathematical thinking in psychologically troubled subjects have been described in detail by Schmid-Kitsikis [1976]. The most important difficulties experienced by such subjects involved exploration of objects and construction of strategies. In exploring objects and relating them to one another, subjects frequently discontinue a search, change criteria for classification, and make personal comments or construct personal scenes with the objects. Their behavior appears disorganized, in contrast to their capacity to determine superordinate classes, which they appear to have abstracted correctly. Their classifying activities appear to be constantly compromised by the influence of associations, contaminations, or perseverations. Corresponding difficulties appear with respect to construction of coherent strategies. Subjects frequently modify their choices and are unsystematic in their sorting behavior. Correction and verification are absent. Often they give up on tasks after a few manipulations.

Our current data confirm and enrich the hypotheses and conclusions of the 1976 work. Our observations show (a) that these subjects have difficulties in regulating their actions, since there is no continuity nor stability in their constructions, and (b) that though constructive activities are not absent, they do not lead to a definite logical structuration, because subjects are led astray by spatio-temporal aspects of their activity, which obstruct the logico-mathematical synchronicity. My interpretation of these subjects' mental functioning is that they attribute to each of their actions a particular causal meaning, which makes creation of the necessary coordinations impossible. Subjects avoid, in particular, the coordination between assimilation and accommodation, and adopt the splitting mechanism, organizing the external world so that it is no longer necessary to make a choice between various possibilities nor to search for equilibrium. The result is a type of destructive negation of thought. This interpretation can also explain a kind of 'filler' activity shown by these subjects, due either to excessive accommodation to reality (spatial contiguities or particular object properties), or to excessive assimilation, which under the influence of the instinctual drives disrupts the links between external and internal reality and creates imaginary or strange objects.

In addition, we notice several behaviors of these subjects that can be interpreted as a renouncement of responsibility for logico-mathematical activity. These subjects often appear to delegate their activity to a person (or an object, or even an event) of their own creation, felt to be all-powerful, so that they themselves can retain the role of director and possessor of knowledge. With the help of these mentally created entities, subjects create intermediary actors with whom they can agree and whose logical thought can be used without feeling any conflict.

This type of functioning shows a desire for a particular equilibrium as a sort of magical absolute. It uses thought and conceptual competence that satisfy an archaic desire for completeness as a source of phantasmic elaborations that safeguard logical competence while sexualizing thought. Thought with this double function (logical and phantasmic) is then believed to dominate both what is good and what is bad, and to create order and harmony in the universe.

Such an analysis of logico-mathemetical activity allows the psychologist to define the problem of the links between primary and secondary processes. Characteristics of the mental functioning of a subject that can be derived from an analysis of behavior in other spheres of thought are confirmed by the investigation of the subject's logico-mathematical activities. The knowledge gained by these activities is the direct product of the organization the subject introduces into his or her actions. In other words, during these activities the object of knowledge is the subject him- or herself. The coordinations of actions thus necessarily refer to the self, whose development depends also on the quality of the libidinal linking forces necessary for the structuring of a thinking subject.

Summary

At the end of this chapter, which, in a way, is the backbone of this volume, it is useful to briefly summarize the psychological meaning of the various mental constructions elaborated by the subject.

With the help of the permanent acquisition of the fundamental invariants, the subject constructs a solid ego.

With the help of representation and the construction of imagined forms, the subject feeds the imagination.

With the help of rational thought, the subject masters the past, the present and the future.

With the help of symbolic substitution, the subject becomes a creator.

These essential constructions provide the subject with access to mental and corporal autonomy, to communication and to creativity.

3

Clinical Applications: Assessment and Treatment

As is usual in clinical consultation, the first analysis concerns the request for consultation itself, and covers the following: (a) the origin of the request (made by the family and/or the school); (b) the interpretation of the request by the psychologist, according to his or her representational system; (c) case history, in order to understand the representations of the subject's parents and of persons in the immediate environment; and (d) the choice of time schedule and venue of the sessions. (This choice can have a favorable or inhibiting influence on the relation to be established between the psychologist and the individuals who come for consultation.)

For this analysis, we take into account both the representations and meanings the psychologist derives from the way the experiential and sociocultural reality of the subject is reported and the actual facts of this reality, though in our experience the latter are only rarely the direct cause of the subject's mental and psychic dysfunction. The manner in which the parents (or the environment) are viewed, desired, and experienced in the child's cognitive and relational functioning is in most cases of greater import than objective reality.

Certain conditions have to be fulfilled for the investigation to be fruitful. The first concerns the role and psychological disposition of the psychologist (his or her relational manner and listening and observing attitude). As already discussed, the psychologist occupies a complex and delicate position in so far as he or she has to be able to combine two attitudes that appear contradictory – a listening attitude that is open to his or her own internal world as well as to the internal world of the subject, and an analyzing attitude that is directed toward observation as well as interpretation. The listening attitude necessitates a kind of 'floating' attention, a mental and psychic availability and relational disposition such that the psychologist can be consciously receptive to the subject's affects, representations, images and ideation. The analyzing attitude necessitates mental alertness, critical reflection, a capacity for forming judgments and a hypothetico-deductive stance. It is necessary to move back and forth between these two attitudes in order to apprehend the affective-cognitive aspects of the subject's psychological organization and functioning, and to manage the psychodynamic situation so as to further the creation of constructive dialectical interactions. The psychologist is thus (depending on the situation) in a position of retreat, on the one hand, since he or she relates to the subject according to what is reactivated in the psychologist's own internal world, and, on the other hand, in a position of active participation in the subject's constructions.

The second set of conditions that have to be fulfilled for fruitful investigation concern definition of the problem. At the first encounter with the subject, the psychologist will already have built up a certain representation, from his or her knowledge of the request (made by an institution, by those responsible for the subject, or by the subject him- or herself), and from any further information collected. The psychologist can either simply use these elements to immediately organize the time and place of sessions, the tasks to be used, etc., or the psychologist may prefer to define his or her own expectations and hypotheses concerning the psychological problems of the subject. Inevitably, our knowledge of the subject's past and the motives for a request for consultation influence our mental and psychic disposition. Though we cannot ignore what we know already, we can voluntarily and provisionally put this knowledge aside, to be used subsequently along with our own discoveries. A request for consultation can be disguised in various ways and to various degrees, and the true meaning of a request or of a piece of information can be understood only if the subject is not immediately inserted into a framework of representations provided by others. A prognosis regarding the subject's psychological development and the construction of a therapeutic plan can be valid only if based on exploration of the subject's psychic and mental characteristics.

The investigation procedures themselves should answer two types of questions. The first concern the subject's acquisitions, what he or she is able to do, to produce and to evoke in a particular situation. The second concern the manner in which the subject tries to solve problems, to interact with the psychologist and with the objects that are present during the session, and to transmit his or her representations. These observations (see Appendix B for a recapitulative and interpretive grid) allow a psychological diagnosis and prognosis.

Theoretical Aspects of Clinical Investigation

I coined the term 'mobilization of mental functioning' to characterize our clinical investigation procedures during which the psychodynamics of the subject are studied with regard to intrapsychic and intra-mental aspects. Though our method is so far used mainly with school-aged children, it can also be used with younger and older subjects (with certain modifications). The fact that in our practice we use both Piagetian and psychoanalytic theory in order to understand the subject distinguishes our method from others.

Certain relational and interactive conditions must be fulfilled if constructive mobilization is to take place. For subjects to be able to discover and to develop their mental capacities with the mental and relational help of the therapist, their capacities for cathexis, for the construction of representational systems, and for the organization of relational activity have to be taken into account. The concept of constructive mobilization is therefore not compatible with other theories that may have similar objectives but use immediately directive methods. Consequently, I shall discuss only psychoanalytic therapeutic methods that use widely known concepts and methods, such as those of A. Freud, Klein and Winnicott, in order to define our own methods more clearly. From this point of view, Winnicott is particularly important because of his focus on the dual relationship between therapist and child, which he sees as evolving inside a 'symbolic space'. In our approach, the dramatic component elicited and shared by the therapist and the subject during the play sessions and interpretive treatment has even greater importance than it does for Winnicott, since it allows an elaboration not only of phantasmic and symbolic activities, but also of relational activities. This component is indeed not absent from Winnicott's work, but it is more often present in psychoanalytic interventions that use the psychodramatic approach [Anzieu, 1985; Wildlocher, 1962; Basquin et al., 1972].

Applications of Piagetian theories to psychotherapy are still rare. They are mostly limited to so-called operatory learning, though in certain cases the authors are guided by the hypothesis that particular learning situations can lead to spreading effects for cognitive functioning in general [Kamii and Devries, 1978; Paour, 1979, 1985, 1987; Orsini-Bouichou, 1982; Orsini-Bouichou and Paour, 1986]. These researchers do not consider cognitive functioning in its relation to libidinal drives (as we do, therefore preferring the term mental to cognitive), and, in general, they ignore the intra-mental dynamics governed by mechanisms such as projective identification, splitting, denial, annulation, projection, introjection, assimilation, accommodation, etc. Their intervention is aimed exclusively at cognitive progress through the mobilization of fundamental operative processes necessary for intelligent activity. The few therapeutic endeavors based on Piagetian theory that exist are illustrated by the procedures developed by Weiner [1975, 1985], who explains that with patients presenting 'deficits or disorganizations of equilibrium' his aim is not so much to reestablish an equilibrium, but rather to develop new psychological structures that will permit a higher-level equilibrium. For Weiner, a Piagetian approach can lead to understanding the reasons for failure, and the quality of the subject's reasoning and emotions that led to the failure. But in order to bring to light an infantile trauma that disturbs psychological equilibrium, the subject's defense mechanisms, as well as his or her retention of certain images and associations during the intellectual task, have to be investigated. This approach leads to two successive stages in the intervention procedure, first an analytical therapy and then an investigation that includes an interpretation of the subject's cognitive functioning and its links to defense mechanisms.

Concerning our own intervention methods, I would emphasize that we do not use Piagetian investigations directly for therapeutic purposes. Their contribution is in allowing the psychologist to apprehend the subject's capacities for change and progress. Since we aim to activate the subject's mental mobility, and thus modify his or her mode of mental functioning, the Piagetian investigations provide us with a foundation and guidelines for effective therapy.

The cathexis process is the most difficult to mobilize or re-mobilize, since it starts at the very beginning of life and leaves its imprint on most spheres of psychological activity. The assimilation mechanism, necessary for mental functioning and for the creation of favorable developmental conditions, depends on cathexes (and countercathexes) and their power of linking libidinal energy. The subject's cognitive activity and the object-to-be-known must be cathected for knowledge to be experienced as meaningful through assimilation. Analysis of the functioning and the organization of the products of assimilation (modulated by accommodation) allows an analysis of the kinds of acquisitions constructed by the subject and, consequently, of the cathectic modes that underlie them. If the subject is to develop favorably, and to be capable of personal elaborations, the constructive process that starts from the undifferentiated and anarchic state of the infant's experiences has to take place under certain relational and interactive conditions, of which the most important is that of psychic and relational continuity. This is why our intervention has to offer the subject the possibility of a continuous relational experience, at the level of the pleasure-displeasure principle as well as at the level of the reality principle, in order to favor discovery, invention and mental creation.

Play situations (in the broad sense) appear particularly well-suited to this objective. They elicit not only verbal communication but also communication in other registers, such as mime, graphics, play-acting, etc. In play, it is possible to observe certain contents of the subject's internal world through his or her phantasmic and symbolic constructions, as well as rational constructions of mental operations that integrate elements of the internal world with the organization of external reality. When play situations are used therapeutically in our approach, they have certain similarities to analytic psychodrama. Indeed, play as an imaginary situation performed theatrically is apt to reveal and to energize certain fantasies in the representation of hidden content [Basquin et al., 1972]. In my view, it is possible to go further and to see play as eliciting constructive mental functioning in the three types of experience that are essential for the subject's psychological development and integration, i.e., emotional, physical, and logico-mathematical experience.

The reader may wonder why I attribute such importance to cognitive constructions as part of therapy. Certain therapists of the psychoanalytic persuasion appear to be guided in their methods by the hypothesis that, at least in the case of children, eventual relational modifications will have a direct generalizing effect on cognitive development and functioning. That this is so seems doubtful, since transference neurosis can lead to an exclusive focus on relational aspects of psychological functioning and a neglect of cognitive aspects (at least for a certain time), and thus endanger the young subject's development. Though periods of construction and reconstruction, of reorganization of functioning (including regressive functioning), certainly occur, they are not, by themselves, sufficient to achieve cognitive compensation. Child psychoanalysts who use only Freudian theory without the contribution of developmental psychology may not be aware of this danger, since they have little interest in the development and enrichment of intellectual capacities.

In contrast, we feel that it is necessary to understand the subject not only as a center for the emergence and activation of phantasmic processes, but also as a center for the development of control strategies, as well as mental anticipation and retroaction. It is for this reason that we have introduced into the therapeutic process various means that both child and therapist can use to construct dramatic scenarios. These include providing objects and suggesting activities such as drawing, cutting, making puppets, constructing stage sets, etc. These activities serve as mediators for the delegation, transposition, and stimulation of representations, and affects, as well as for substitution strategies and discovery procedures. We thus offer children a space for relations and realizations they can undertake (if they want to and are psychologically able to do so) in order to express their many-sidedness: to put what is internal somewhere external, to put inside oneself something that is outside, to live and let live, to construct and let be constructed, to be and to do, and to observe as well as to participate.

Definition of Our Intervention Methods and of Their Links with Child Psychoanalysis and Individual Analytic Psychodrama[1]

The psychologist or psychoanalyst who works within a psychodynamic framework needs to analyze the problems that underlie the subject's observable symptoms. This task is common to all such therapeutic intervention, but the elements that enter into the diagnosis and the way it is undertaken vary considerably with the theoretical approach. The traditional psychoanalytic approach draws on interviews with the child and the parents, and activities such as play and drawing, and focuses on the subject's intrapsychic world as it may be apprehended via the history of sexuality, representations, and ego cathexes. Our own approach, as indicated earlier, aims at a diagnosis of the mental functioning of the subject in its affective-cognitive aspects, through analysis of the relation the subject establishes between his or her interior reality and external reality. Compared to psychoanalysts, we thus accord much greater importance to the evaluation of the subject's capacities to deal with reality in the here-and-now.

In individual psychodramatic therapy, the subject is in the presence of two therapists, one of each sex. In our work we use the dyadic situation customary in psychoanalysis. Sometimes a group situation is used, three therapists and one child [Schmid-Kitsikis and Weinstein, 1983]. The spac-

[1] Parts of the following analysis derive from the work of N. Fuchs, a graduate student who worked under my direction.

ing of sessions is the same as in psychodramatic therapy, i.e., once a week, whereas in psychoanalysis sessions are more frequent, usually four or five times a week.

The duration of therapy can be determined either by a contract in which the number of sesssions is specified from the beginning or by the progress as it is absorbed and analyzed from one session to the next. In general we prefer a comparatively short duration, and this is often possible when the therapist analyzes and interprets in detail the data collected before the first session as well as after each completed session.

Concerning the use of materials during therapeutic sessions, we differ from those who work in the psychodramatic tradition. The latter regard the presence of accessory objects as a hindrance to pretense; even if the child brings toys to the session, the therapist will put them aside. In our view, there is no reason to attribute an unfavorable role to objects. All objects have manifold meanings, not simply one particular social value, and it is precisely the various representations the objects elicit in the subject that are of interest. It is true of course that the object influences the way the child is going to use it. For those of the psychoanalytic school, both the number and types of objects must be carefully chosen. In our work we use simple objects, such as pieces of wood, string, paper, yogurt cartons, nutshells, corks, etc., which can be employed in various ways and which the child can use for graphic activities, and modeling, and that can be talked about and used in symbolic play [Schmid-Kitsikis, 1985a, p. 102]. The use the child makes of these objects informs the therapist about their covert meanings, the phantasmic contents they evoke, and their constructions and modes of elaboration. In so far as possible, the objects introduced should not carry precise social connotations that lead to fixed roles in play, limiting the imagination and spontaneity of the child.

Therapeutic Organization of the Session

In psychodramatic play, sessions are divided into two segments – first the child's proposals for a theme and for the distribution of different roles, and then the 'mise en scène' by the participants who will act in the play. The duration of the psychodramatic play is usually ten minutes, but it may be shortened if there are signs of the child's acting out. The implicit criterion is that of pretense, acting as if; if this criterion is not adhered to, the therapist may terminate the activity. The play should have a beginning and an end during the same session. As soon as a theme has appeared in the child's play, the therapist suggests modifications and variations. Freedom in the play session may thus be restricted. This may be necessary when, 'because of the intensity of emotional discharge, a continuation of the play session could minimize its incisive character; the objective pursued is not to find meanings via associations, but to stop when what has to be said has indeed been expressed' [Basquin et al., 1972, p. 26, translated from original].

No explicit conditions concerning temporal organization are imposed in psychoanalytic sessions. Generally, the analyst endeavors to elicit associations, though exceptions may occur (e.g., when a child begins to act destructively, the analyst may intervene by other than interpretive means). No particular sequence is mandatory with respect to play activities, dream narrations, etc.

Our therapeutic sessions are similar to analytic sessions in this last respect. Apart from the predetermined 45-minute total period, there is no rigid division into segments of a certain duration. We do, however, try to establish a phase during which the theme is decided by means of negotiation between child and therapist, a phase during which objects are chosen and scenarios are planned, and finally a phase during which the play itself is acted out. The elaboration of a theme and the necessary preparation can start during one session and continue during the next. Material constructed during one session is kept in a box (if the child so desires) and provided at the next session.

In comparison to sessions conducted within a psychodramatic or psychoanalytic framework, our sessions have the following characteristics:

(1) The phase of elaborating a theme and the play itself are not necessarily separated (as in psychodramatic sessions), but during play the theme can be further developed and changed. A sequence of (a) theme proposals, (b) negotiations between child and therapist, and (c) actual play, is not a necessary condition but reflects a satisfactory evolution of the treatment.

(2) The elaboration of a theme as a story to be worked out can span several sessions and thus encourage the subject to maintain certain mental representations established earlier.

(3) The therapist not only encourages the subject to make associations but also promotes their insertion into a sequence that presents certain logical links (in contrast to the analytic approach).

Modes of Expression in Play

In our own as well in psychoanalytic and psychodramatic approaches, play occupies a central position. Psychodramatically and analytically, play is considered to reveal unconscious conflicts and thus, within the therapeutic relation, to provide occasion for the expression, construction and reconstruction of the subject's internal world (its contents and the way they are experienced), by way of the subject's phantasmic and symbolic elaborations. Though the aim of all three approaches, i.e., the mobilization of the subject's psychic and mental potentialities, is the same, we pay attention also to the socio-cognitive aspects of communication, as they appear during play. Like Kleinian theorists, we believe that the mode of mental functioning apt to lead to further development includes a certain capacity on the part of the subject to confront his or her fantasies with reality; in our situation this confrontation takes place in the here-and-now of the session. All expressive means used by the subject (gestures, mime, drawings, manipulation of objects) are taken into account, even more than verbal expression, since actions represent, physically, spatiotemporally and rationally, the relations the subject establishes between the internal and the external world.

In contrast, in psychodramatic sessions, gestures and verbal expressions are the only actions considered necessary for the actualization of pretense. All other actions are prohibited, especially while the stage is being set. Moreover, in this approach the capacity for symbolization is considered as a necessary condition for undertaking the treatment. In our method, by contrast, it is often a result of the treatment, leading to further mental development. In view of our aim to create a symbolic space (in Winnicott's sense), the introduction of objects into the play situation is an important feature, since they can provide a symbolic support for fantasy and a means for mediating relations.

Interpretation of Play

During child psychoanalysis, interpretation, considered at the level of transfer, is transmitted verbally. It is inspired by observation of the child's play, which is (especially since Klein's discoveries) seen as the substitute par excellence for adult associations. The interpretation is given by the analyst outside of the play situation, so that, even if play and interpretation are closely linked, they take place at different times.

Both the nature and timing of interpretation are different in our approach. We do not explicitly refer to the child's sexual history. Rather, the spontaneous response of the therapist (which is in fact the result of long training), whether verbal or motoric, will lead the subject to link, to feel and to give meaning to the contents and affects expressed, by means of the analyst's own representations, understanding and feelings in relation to the child and in the here-and-now of the session(s). These responses are expressed as part of the play situation, thus making it possible for meanings to be attributed through acting rather than through talking. In this respect, our technique is closer to the psychodramatic approach than the psychoanalytic. The therapist takes the latent meanings of the child's expressions into account and relates them to the reality principle during play. Psychoanalytic interpretation, by contrast, is focused on the unconscious, with its atemporal character and its distorted and distorting representations. Such interpretation ignores the socio-cognitive aspect central to our approach, an aspect which, in a way, may be considered more limited as well as more extensive.

Transference and Countertransference

In psychoanalysis, projections are made only on the analyst. In the psychodramatic situation, the subject is confronted with two therapists (of different sex) who constitute the target for the subject's projections, fantasies and unconscious desires. Both the presence of two therapists and the instructions given (tell each of us what role to play and invent a theme) invite the subject in a direct way to projection and transference.

Our technique is similar to the psychoanalytic one in this respect, but the presence of objects that can be used in the play situation elicits various projections and representations. As in the psychoanalytic situation, these can be interpreted as a resurgence of parental imagos, but other analyses are possible, due to the socio-cognitive aspects of the situation. Since the therapist in the course of the play sessions performs actions with objects and plays various roles, thus evoking in the subject preconscious and conscious images and representations of physical and social aspects of the real world, many different unconscious elaborations are activated in the subject.

In all three psychotherapeutic methods, the therapist must adopt attitudes of listening and discovering. This fundamental similarity apart, there are important differences, especially concerning countertransference mechanisms. In adult psychoanalysis, the so-called attitude of benevolent neutrality of the analyst incites countertransference (as a factor that inhibits transference and identification) and implies that the analyst is only present through interpretations. In child psychoanalysis, the active, motoric participation of the analyst is also reduced to a minimum. The analyst's role is thus essentially that of an observer, whose 'floating attention' creates a space for the mental elaboration necessary for formulation of interpretations, for example concerning transference.

By contrast, in the psychodramatic approach, as well as in our own technique, the therapist assumes a more spontaneous and participating role. In both the latter methods the expression of countertransference is more direct and the variety of possibilities for adjustment is greater. Benevolent neutrality cannot be maintained, but mental activity benefits from greater liberty. The scenarios created by therapist and child, the action sequences that necessitate a certain rationality in our method, as well as the psychodramatic aspect of the therapeutic alliance, facilitate and stimulate the projections and identifications of the child in both an affective and cognitive context.

In contrast to the psychoanalyst's benevolent neutrality, the therapist in our method fulfills both a 'receptive' and a 'constructive' role. Though the methods imply these dissimilarities, they are not contradictory.

A Clinical Example: Stéphane

Stéphane came for consultation at the age of 9. A few months earlier he had become a student at a so-called 'active' school, and his teacher found his scholastic achievement poor. The teacher also noticed that Stéphane only rarely managed to finish a task, that he seemed incapable of organizing his work over the school week, and that he easily panicked when faced with a task he thought too difficult. Stéphane also appeared to have difficulties in becoming part of a group, and often seemed to sulk on his own. His teacher suggested our consultation service to Stéphane's mother.

From interviewing the mother, we obtained the following information. From the age of 18 months, Stéphane was enrolled in various day-care centers, as his mother was professionally active. Stéphane first encountered difficulties at the end of second grade (age 8), when his teacher contacted a municipal service. Stéphane's mother accepted an interview with the service and Stéphane went there for a few sessions, but his mother soon stopped the consultations. At the end of the next school year, Stéphane was once again failing, with the possibility of having to repeat the grade. To avoid this, his mother transferred Stéphane to the 'active' school.

During our interview with Stéphane's mother, she several times expressed her desire for her son to assume responsibility; and, indeed, Stéphane tries to adopt the role of an adult, particularly in his relationship with his younger sister. Stéphane's mother is perfectly content with her daughter, but feels disappointed in her son, who, according to her, only rarely is independent and successful. The family situation changed some years ago, when the parents separated and the father went back to his own country in the Middle-East, where the children visit him at regular intervals. The departure of the father and onset of Stéphane's difficulties in school seem to have coincided.

Stéphane seems preoccupied with the relation between his parents, who apparently have not yet decided whether they will divorce or reconcile. Stéphane is unable to establish parental references and imagos, and is torn between his desire to create a positive image of his father and the negative image of the absent spouse he receives from his mother. Similarly, Stéphane is confronted with the contradiction between his desire to adapt to the reality of the moment and his wish to retrieve the worry-free period of his early childhood. (He searches for objects and pictures of this period and asks questions about his birth and conception.) His mother interprets Stéphane's behavior in this respect as a desire for a return to the family unit, 'a sort of golden age' as she calls it.

Mental Functioning and Competencies

During our first session, Stéphane appeared lively, intelligent and quick to adapt; but he also appeared tense and preoccupied. His intellectual achievements are in general congruent with his age group, both in logico-mathematical reasoning and in spatial organization, though Stéphane approaches problems in a roundabout way, using procedures that are costly in time and energy. He often uses step-by-step reasoning, with many ramifications and without a clear direction. Often, Stéphane begins a task without even listening to the instructions and indulges in much disorganized trial-and-error behavior. His fear of being unable to answer questions leads him to reverse his own role and that of the psychologist: he responds to questions with questions of his own. Yet he is quite capable of taking advantage of the psychologist's suggestions. Stéphane is interested in the problem and would like to find the solution.

All along, Stéphane tries to limit his exchanges with the psychologist to a minimum, as if every personal contact is felt to be intrusive. Stéphane tries to control the psychologist, as he tries to control objects of knowledge. He is most at ease in task situations in which there occur observable, verifiable events. This tendency seems to correspond to his interest in technical matters and particularly computers, a task area in which he excels; indeed, when working with computers Stéphane can avoid the difficulties he has with interpersonal contacts.

Indications for Psychotherapy

Stéphane's desire to control both the relational object and the object of knowledge indicates that he has cathected his mental activity and that he aspires to knowledge (even if this desire for knowledge is for the moment limited to its empirical and technical aspects). Though Stéphane is clearly afraid of failure as well as of contacts with others, he is able to benefit from suggestions made by the psychologist. Stéphane appears to possess a relatively well-established ego, he can function symbolically at a primary and secondary level, and thus it seems possible to enlarge his field of interest. The main objective of our intervention is the discovery by Stéphane of the pleasure that can be derived from personal creations shared with the therapist, and the integration of Stéphane's imaginative world and his rational world, thus permitting him to insert his affects into his mental functioning, instead of excluding them.

An Example of Play Sessions[2]

In the first session, Stéphane explores our material and chooses a ping-pong ball which he lets roll down a wooden slope, and which, in answer to one of my questions, he identifies as a skier. We then decide to construct a mountain village with its inhabitants. Several sessions are taken up with thinking out the scenario and deciding the roles of the main actors: There will be an architect, called Monsieur Dupont (made by myself from a pine cone, with pipe cleaners for arms and legs, and a ball of paper for a head), whose role I will take, and an imaginary person called Jim, whose role Stéphane will take. Jim does not have physical representation, but Stéphane establishes Jim as a driver of cars and pilot of airplanes and speaks for Jim when necessary. Sometimes Stéphane also plays other characters (made by myself) and integrates them into the story we create together. We build a village, with houses, a church, a park, a restaurant, using wooden blocks, modelling clay and bits of plastic. In later sessions, a school is built, and several events, either in a family, in school, or in a recreation park are enacted.

The play space becomes gradually wider and more cathected by Stéphane. He then expresses the desire to explore new regions: We build the New York airport in a corner. The director of the airport (called Bob Barnett and played by myself) makes friends with the villagers. Jim goes to the airport to demonstrate his new prototype airplane. Barnett places an order and the two become associates and conduct excursions by car and by plane. Stéphane decides to construct a secret submarine base in another corner. Only the villagers know of its existence, and only they have right of access. Stéphane constructs this base on his own: He makes a submarine, an amphibious car, some robots, and a control tower (with complex, realistic adjuncts). The village remains the point of reference and starting point for various excursions (by helicopter, balloon, car, etc.). The temporal sequence of events is coherent. Indeed, Stéphane seems to attach great importance to the coherence and rationality of our activities. When I propose building a bridge over the runway, as a shortcut to the village, Stéphane opposes the idea and proposes a road with traffic lights for the security of the villagers and as an unobstructed runway for the planes.

Stéphane has no difficulty in narrating the rational and spatial aspects of the setting, but in the beginning he neglects the temporal links between events. All events seem to happen in the immediate present, without any consideration of the future (plan for or anticipation of coming events), nor of the time it will take to carry out certain actions or to

[2] Stéphane's therapy was carried out by Vesna Cvjetanovic (one of my collaborators) and supervised by myself. The description of the sessions was written by the therapist.

prepare for them. All is practically finished before it has begun, as if everything should be done before it can be thought out. The time of day is not defined, and the planes defy time by crossing the ocean in seconds. Little by little Stéphane begins to take time into account. During the 14th session, Jim (Stéphane) refuses to discuss the construction of a school with the architect, and immediately gathers the necessary material as well as a schoolbus and a plane. But then he announces that night has fallen and that it is time to go to bed. The villagers go to sleep, and Jim telephones the architect. Together they decide to prepare a surprise for the villagers when they wake up in the morning. Stéphane then emits a 'cock-a-doodle-doo' to signal the passage of time. A new day begins. Gradually time and space become integrated into the play.

At the 16th session, as soon as he arrives, Stéphane reconstructs the village on the floor, in haste, but using only the objects he made or used himself, and leaves me seated at the table with mine. Playing the role of the architect, I remark that Jim seems to have decided to live elsewhere and that the village seems to be rather empty. At first Stéphane continues his activity, but then he interrrupts it, looks intently at me and declares, 'You know, I have left the village because I'm told that I am champion of inventions, but I don't want people to come and get me to make inventions in their country'. The architect responds, 'Maybe you think that they will ask you to make something so complex that you can't be sure of getting it right'. Stéphane replies, 'Even so, I'm not interested in money ... but they could ask me to make bad things, like an atomic bomb'. The architect says, 'You think that they may ask you to make dangerous things and you don't know how to refuse; so you prefer to hide yourself.' Stéphane is worried: 'But they could come and threaten me with a gun and make me do it.' He then constructs a sort of frame with pipe cleaners and asks me to guess what it is. I say, 'It looks like a shelter.' Stéphane smiles and says, 'You got it.' Then the architect asks where Jim is. 'I am under the water,' answers Stéphane, and the architect adds that maybe Jim feels better hidden and more protected under water. Stéphane says that he will visit the village and build himself a house there. The architect can then come and visit him whenever he likes. The architect remarks, 'You feel rather lonely, I suppose.' Stéphane answers sadly that he is very busy with his constructions. 'Yes, but you have no company,' says the architect. Stéphane is worried but defends himself (with little conviction): 'Sometimes there are people passing by. Yesterday I saw a submarine and I waved to the people inside'. He smiles a little. The architect decides to pay Jim a visit with his son, as Jim invited him to do. The first thing Jim wants to know is how the villagers are doing. The architect tells him that the villagers send their greetings and that they often think of Jim.

In the few minutes before the end of the session, Stéphane begins to move the things he displaced in the opposite direction. The architect wonders, 'Maybe Jim is afraid that the villagers will be angry if he doesn't come back'. Stéphane quickly puts everything back in the village and says, 'No, it's like you said before. I don't want to be alone over there.'

During the last session, I had the feeling that Stéphane was far more open to dialogue, that he even wanted me to discuss his feelings, as if only verbal explicitness could bring appeasement. In the beginning of the therapy, Stéphane was busy building and played different roles and hardly expressed his feelings, remaining on the defensive (sometimes even taking the offensive) whenever I dared to comment on our exchanges and the emotions we felt when we acted our parts. Our verbal exchanges about various emotional matters only gradually acquired the same relational value as our shared constructions, stories or telephone conversations.

Comments

It is necessary for the therapist to take into account the different spheres of mental functioning of the subject, the cognitive as well as the emotional. The therapist's interventions and responses to the subject's actions or utterances thus cover a wide field. The responses take the form of material actions (constructing objects) or creative and rational productions (narration of a story or actual event), social and interactive exchanges (dialogues between the partners in the play concerning the reality they deal with) and relational exchanges (verbalizations of what seems to happen inside the subject on the relational level).

In the sessions described above, my interpretations established links between what was happening at the moment (impressions of sadness, solitude, and fear, of 'doing bad things' expressed by Stéphane) with what happened in earlier sessions. My aim was to create a continuity, i.e., a relational and psychic continuity, a continuity of meanings, and a sociohistorical continuity. Thus, when Stéphane performed an action (a move away from the village), the architect (myself) expressed, as an inhabitant of the village, a feeling of loss. Stéphane often play-acted scenes that touched on his father's absence and his own incapacity to find his father again, but usually such episodes led to a desire for omnipotence that eliminated all feelings of sadness and solitude, whereas in this last session Stéphane's feelings were expressed. Similarly, this time Stéphane expressed his desire to protect himself against the bad things he might do and he built a shelter (an atomic shelter), thus giving material form to what was expressed verbally. He is also capable of going inside his submarine base and feeling abandoned and anxious. Instead of indulging in excessive activity or creating all-powerful magical thoughts, Stéphane can experience and symbolize his geographical displacement and his fear of being forgotten or losing his proximity to me if he remains absent for too long (identification with what he experienced with his father and his mother).

By transmitting back to Stéphane the feelings of solitude, sadness and fear he made me experience, I could make him accept these feelings as his own. These interpretations concerned particularly the emotions felt by Stéphane in the relation of transference. At other times I also intervened at the level of social interaction and in the process of autonomization.

To conclude, the central issue in therapy is, in our view, that of the connections between developments in different spheres, i.e., of object relations and of cognitive energies, as well as the quality of the mental constructions and acquisitions that are already present. There are certainly therapeutic methods that, for subjects with deficiencies, improve their relational capacities and their social interaction, or that increase their learning abilities. But as far as we know, there is no therapeutic method that combines these different objectives into an integrated whole, allowing the therapist to make regular progress and ensure success. Though our own method aims to mobilize the subject's mental capacities, it does not necessarily have a direct effect on intellectual performance. We can prepare a subject's mental functioning for intellectual learning, but we do not monitor new acquisitions (or, at least, we do not establish a framework for doing so).

The theoretical and methodological positions outlined in this chapter focus on conditions that favor the mobilization in subjects of existing, but insufficiently exploited, forces, in order to enable them to take charge of their own mental development. Clearly, this approach could be enriched by methods aimed at promoting intellectual attitudes that would enable subjects to take charge of their own cognitive achievements.

4

Summary and Conclusions

In this volume I have tried, through an integrative approach, to examine a variety of different aspects of mental functioning and to explore the interaction between components of mental functioning that are usually studied separately. Indeed, my principal hypothesis concerns the necessity of an integration between conceptual and emotional thought. In other words, I propose that, for thought to be truly creative, it must remain open to primary processes, even though it functions predominantly in terms of secondary processes. Analysis of the various modes of mental functioning of both 'well-adapted' and 'marginal' subjects provides relevant data within this theoretical framework, particularly concerning the relations between the different processes of representation. Indeed, symbolic functioning constitutes in my opinion an intersection between the different mental functions and their modes of construction. It takes its material from conscious, preconscious and/or unconscious elements and plays its part in various ways both in rational and in imaginative thinking.

In a clinical context, the tasks we use as practicing psychologists make it possible to observe subjects' ability to realize their cognitive-affective potentialities in a particular situation with its temporal limitations: the psychological interview. Subjects attach a certain meaning to this situation. There is a necessity for relational adjustment since conflicts may emerge or be activated by the psychologist, and the significance of certain behaviors, particularly their mobility and variety, can be assessed. From a clinical point of view, the psychological interview situation permits the psychologist to construct a relationship with the subject, to elicit certain unconscious processes that are related to the subject's desires, motivations and behavior. The relations that are established between the psychologist and the subject mobilize a certain affective economy and various representational systems with their complex cathexes that go far beyond the particular hic et nunc situations.

Our therapeutic intervention aims at the mobilization of whatever mental potentialities the subject possesses. The various situations demand of the subject different ways of 'being together' with the therapist and make it possible to develop the quality and nature of object relations under the influence of drive energy and its representations. The different ways of 'being together' within a relational context lead to representations, symbolizations and rationalizations of thoughts about external reality, as well as about one's self.

The particular temporal conditions of therapeutic situations offer opportunities for our understanding of different levels of representation, especially if the therapist solicits the subject's emotional, relational and social, as well as cognitive, capacities. In a sense, the importance I accord at a theoretical level to the integration of these various capacities within an individual's mental functioning parallels what for the psychologist must be a constant endeavor to integrate theoretical considerations with clinical observations and applications.

Appendix A

Tasks

This appendix contains a description of tasks used in our practice. The tasks described are grouped in four categories (A, B, C, D), though certain tasks may be considered to belong to two or more categories. The primary grouping is based on the tasks' main characteristics and their clinical interest. The links of a task to other categories are indicated. The description of the tasks does not cover the relational and interactional conditions of our clinical approach (these are treated in Chapter 2); the emphasis is on their technical aspects. The procedures of the Piagetian tasks (described in detail since they may be less familiar to clinical psychologists than other tasks) closely follow the technique described in the original works, but show certain adaptations and modifications introduced for clinical application. (Only the adaptations for use with children are indicated.)

In general, use of these tasks call for interview conditions that allow the main objective to be focused, and a system of protocol notation that permits a detailed analysis of the subject's behavior and discovery procedure. The Piagetian approach aims at the establishment of a 'natural' dialogue between subject and psychologist and the creation of a social context, as the psychologist confronts subjects with opinions supposedly expressed by their peers. In our practice, we emphasize the need to avoid a situation in which the subject is placed in direct confrontation with a psychologist who expresses counterarguments. It is preferable for the psychologist to play the part of an arbiter who negotiates between two subjects expressing different opinions.

Since most Piagetian tasks do not readily lend themselves to standardization, we simply indicate the age range for which the task is clinically interesting.

Category A
The Construction of Invariants

Task A1. The Construction of Numerical Equivalence or One-to-One Correspondence

Reference: Piaget, J. & Inhelder, B. Structures numériques élémentaires, ECG, vol. XIII: 19 (Presses Universitaires de France, Paris, 1962); Piaget, J. & Szeminska A. La genèse du nombre chez l'enfant, chap. III: 69–77 (Delachaux & Niestlé, 1941 Neuchâtel); translated into English (1952) as: *The child's conception of number.* Atlantic Highlands: The Humanities Press.

Materials: 12 red and 12 blue counters (or 12 eggs and 12 egg cups).

Procedure: 7 red counters (egg cups) are aligned (2 centimeters apart).

Item 1: The subject is asked to put down as many (just as many, the same number of) blue counters (eggs), as red no more, no less. The subject is left free to manipulate the counters till s/he declares that s/he has finished. The psychologist then asks: What did you do? Are there just as many blue counters as red ones? How do you know? Could you explain it to somebody else? Why do you think there are just as many? The task proceeds to item 2 when the subject has established a correct one-to-one correspondence. If this cannot be achieved, the psychologist establishes the correspondence and asks the subject whether there is the same number, or continues the task starting from an inequality if the subject appears to want this.

Item 2: The subject is asked to put the red counters (egg cups) close together, without spaces between them (if necessary, the psychologist does it) and the psychologist asks: And now are there just as many (the same number) of red counters (egg cups) as blue ones (eggs)? How do you know? Can you explain? If the subject says that there are not the same number, s/he is asked: What should we do so that there are again just as many? the same number? If the subject does not respond, the interviewer asks: Can we add some more there? (pointing to the row where the subject thinks there are less) *or* Can we take away some from there? (pointing to the row where the subject thinks there are more).

In order to evaluate the solidity of the subject's answers, the psychologist proposes a counterargument in the form of a fictive dialogue: You know, somebody said (repeating what the subject said) ... and somebody else didn't agree, s/he said ... If the subject does not change his/her answer, the psychologist can go further: You see, he said that there was the same number because no counters were taken away or added, but the other one still said there were more here, because the row goes further ... What do you think? Who is right? If the subject changes his/her answers, one or several items of the task are repeated.[1]

Age range: 3 to 7 years.

[1] All the tasks in this group are to be concluded by this kind of counterargumentation. Since it always takes the same general form, it will not be described for the other tasks.

Task A2. One-to-One Exchange: Playing Shop

Reference: Piaget, J. & Szeminska A. La genèse du nombre chez l'enfant, chap. III: 77–82 (Delachaux & Niestlé, 1941 Neuchâtel); translated into English (1952) as: *The child's conception of number.* Atlantic Highlands: The Humanities Press.

Materials: 9 pennies, 12 small packages, a basket.

Procedure: Psychologist and subject play shop.

Item 1: The subject is the client. The subject is told: You take the money and go shopping. I am the shopkeeper and each time you buy a package you give me a penny. Each package costs a penny. When the subject has bought 9 packages, there are 3 left which are put aside. The psychologist holds the pennies in his or her hand and asks: Have I got just as many pennies as you have packages, or have I more pennies, or you more packages? If the subject has difficulties, the psychologist asks whether it would help to look at the packages to find out how many coins the shopkeeper has in his or her hand.

Item 2: The subject plays the role of the shopkeeper. The same questions are asked. Sometimes the psychologist suggests that this time the subject ask the questions.

Item 3: The psychologist is again the client. After the sixth package has been bought and the shopkeeper still has 6 packages left, the psychologist asks: Do you know how many pennies I still have in my hand? After two more buys, the psychologist asks the same question once again. After all the packages have been bought, the psychologist asks: With all the pennies you have now, could you buy all these packages? Could you buy more? Do you have enough for all the packages?

Age range: 3 to 6 years (With the youngest subjects, fewer packages are used).

Note: This task is particularly interesting from the relational and interactional point of view.

Task A3. Conservation of Liquids

Reference: Piaget, J. & Szeminska, A. La genèse du nombre chez l'enfant, chap. I: 16–42 (Delachaux & Niestlé, 1941 Neuchâtel); translated into English (1952) as: *The child's conception of number.* Atlantic Highlands: The Humanities Press.

Materials: 2 identical glasses, A and A′ (about 5 cm in diameter and 8 cm tall); one narrower and taller glass, N (about 3 cm in diameter and 12 cm tall); one wider, shorter glass, W (about 7 cm in diameter and 4 cm tall); 4 identical little glasses each about one fourth of the volume of A –L1, L2, L3 and L4; 2 bottles containing colored water (e.g., one red and one green).

Procedure: The psychologist first gets the subject to agree that A and A′ are the same size. S/he then pours water (or juice) into A and asks the subject to take the other bottle and to pour the same amount into A′: Pour exactly the same amount, no more no less. If the subject finds the pouring too difficult, the psychologist can do it instead asking the subject to say 'stop' when there is the same amount in both glasses. When the subject agrees that both have the same amount, the task starts. If no agreement can be reached, the task can be carried out on unequal amounts (the inequality then has to be conserved).

Item 1: The psychologist says that the juice from glass A will be poured into glass N and then asks: How far up will the juice go, do you think? Will there be just as much juice to drink in glass A and glass N? The psychologist then pours the juice from glass A to glass N and observes whether the subject is surprised. The subject is asked: Did you think it would go up like that? Whatever the answer, the psychologist then asks: Do we both have just as much to drink? Or does one of us have more? How do you know? How could you explain it to somebody else? If the subject gives a nonconservation answer, the psychologist asks: What should we do so that we have the same amount to drink? It is made clear that the subject can add or take away liquid. Then the subject is asked: And now, if I pour the juice from N to A, how far up will the juice go? Will there be as much juice in A as in N? How can you explain it? The liquid is then poured back into A, and the same questions are asked as in the beginning. If necessary, the amounts may be readjusted so that the subject agrees that there is equality.

Item 2: The liquid is poured from A′ into W. The interview is carried out as in item 1.

Item 3: The liquid is poured from A′ to L1, L2, L3 and L4 . (The 4 small glasses should contain about the same amount of liquid.) The interview is carried out as for the first two items, making it clear that the comparison bears on the liquid in A and that the question concerns the liquid contained in all the 4 small glasses taken together.

Variations: If a subject above the age of 6 or 7, by which time a child is expected to have acquired the conservation concept, is unable to give conservation answers, the psychologist presents once again the different items and asks the subject each time to add or take away juice so that there is the same amount, and then the liquid is immediately poured back into the original glass. If the subject is aware of the difference (in level and amount), once again the psychologist requests: Make it so that it is the same. If indeed the subject adds or takes away some liquid (which happens frequently) the psychologist starts with smaller amounts in A and A′, so that after pouring into differently shaped glasses the levels are not very different. (Sometimes the subject then accepts that there is still the same amount: I saw that we needed almost all the juice [in N] for it to be the same.)

Age range: 3 to 8 years.

Task A4. Conservation of Quantity of Matter

Reference: Piaget, J. & Inhelder, B. Le développement des quantités chez l'enfant, chap. I: 6–29 (Delachaux & Niestlé, 1941 Neuchâtel); translated into English (1974) as: *The child's construction of quantities. Conservation and atomism.* New York: Basic Books.

Materials: 2 balls of modelling clay of 2 different colors.

Procedure: The psychologist says: I have two balls of clay. I want there to be as much in the one as in the other, just the same (same amount, just as much). If there is a difficulty for the child in establishing equality of the matter contained in the 2 balls, the psychologist can suggest some edible material (pastry dough) and ask the questions in terms of 'getting just as much to eat'. If the subject does not admit equality, the task can be carried out starting from inequality.

Item 1: The psychologist asks the child to change the shape of one of the balls into that of a rather thin sausage. (If the child has difficulties, the psychologist does it.) Then the following questions are asked: Is there just as much playdough in the ball as in the sausage? Or is there more in the ball or more in the sausage? The psychologist also asks for justifications and arguments. If the subject gives nonconservation answers, the psychologist continues: If I remake the sausage into a ball, how will it be? Will there be as much clay in the one ball as in the other? Or more in one of them? If necessary, readjustments are made so that the child agrees to the equality.

Item 2: One of the balls is transformed into a pancake (cookie). The interview proceeds as in item 1.

Item 3: One of the balls is cut into little bits. The interview then proceeds as in item 2. The psychologist should make it clear that the questions about quantity bear on a comparison between all the bits, on the one hand, and the ball, on the other.

Other transformations can be presented (ring, bowl, snake) in order to clarify the subject's difficulties and bring to light eventual discordances. In general it is important to note the fluctuations, oscillations, compromises, etc., and the arguments given by the subject.

Variations: (1) The psychologist asks the subject to perform the transformation slowly, and to pay attention to the form of the object by feeling it with his or her hands. The psychologist may ask the subject to flatten the ball with one hand, and to use the other hand to trace its dimensions. (Several successive small transformations are to be performed.) After each small transformation, the question of the quantity is asked. Then the subject is asked to perform the inverse transformation, back to the ball, again in small steps. The subject is asked to foresee what will happen when the ball is reconstituted: same amount? more or less? If the subject's reasoning appears to improve, the psychologist returns to the original procedure.

(2) The psychologist presents 3 balls, A, B and C, of equal size. The subject is asked to transform the ball B a bit towards a sausage, whereupon the psychologist transforms C somewhat more towards the sausage-shape, and so on. The subject is then asked to compare A and B, B and C, and A and C at different stages of the transformation process. This variation allows the psychologist to observe transitivity reasoning on the part of the subject. The effects of these variations should be checked by presenting different transformations of a shape. The variations are particularly interesting with subjects who give nonconservation answers in the traditional version of the tasks.

Age range: 5 to 9 years.

Task A5. Conservation of Weight

Reference: Piaget, J. & Inhelder, B. Le développement des quantités chez l'enfant, chap. II: 30–59 (Delachaux & Niestlé, 1941 Neuchâtel); translated into English (1974) as: *The child's construction of quantities. Conservations and atomism.* New York: Basic Books.

Materials: A balance (weighing instrument formed of two dishes hanging from a beam supported in the middle), 2 balls of modelling clay of different color and of approximately the same weight.

Procedure: The psychologist must ascertain that the subject understands how the balance works; objects of different weight should be available in order to demonstrate the horizontality of the beam and the equal distance of the dishes from the table when two objects (e.g., a key and a lump of modelling clay, which can be adjusted) have the same weight or not. Then the subject is asked to make two balls of the same weight. The psychologist notes how the subject proceeds – by adding, taking away, compressing, etc. If the subject cannot constitute two balls of equal weight, the procedure starts from an inequality (which may or may not be conserved).

Items 1, 2 and 3 are identical to those for the conservation of quantity of matter, but before asking the questions about weight, the psychologist moves the two shapes toward the dishes of the balance and asks the child to anticipate 'how they will be'. If the child gives a nonconservation answer s/he is asked to 'make them so that they weigh the same'. After some transformations, the psychologist may actually put the shapes on the balance, noting whether the subject is surprised. It is also useful to check on the possible effect of the position of the shapes on the dish by transforming one of the balls into a long 'snake' whose head and tail hang down over the dish, or on the effect of visual impressions, such as a transformation into a ring whose circumference seems less important than the big hole in the middle.

Variations: The variations described for the conservation of quantity of matter can also be used for the conservation of weight.

Note: It is sometimes difficult to discern whether subjects are arguing about quantity of matter or about weight. The psychologist should ask the child to elaborate vague expressions ('it's the same') and insist on the act of weighing and on the function of the balance. (If necessary the psychologist uses the child's vocabulary and tries to introduce distinctions such as fat/heavy, big/heavy, etc.)

Age range: 6 to 10 years.

Task A6. Conservation of Volume

Reference: Piaget, J. & Inhelder, B. Le développement des quantités chez l'enfant, chap. II: 60–79 (Delachaux & Niestlé, 1941 Neuchâtel); translated into English (1974) as: *The child's construction of quantities. Conservation and atomism.* New York: Basic Books.

Materials: 2 balls of clay; one metal ball the same size as the clay balls; 2 identical glasses; 2 elastic rubber bands.

Procedure: The subject is asked to fill the 2 glasses with water up to the same level, and to observe that the 2 clay balls are 'the same'. The psychologist then proposes to put the rubber bands around the glasses exactly where the water level is and asks: If I put this ball into one of the glasses of water, what will happen? After the subject indicates what s/he expects, the psychologist immerses the ball, and notes whether the subject is surprised. If the subject anticipates that the water will go up, the psychologist asks, before actually immersing the ball, why this should be so. Otherwise, this question is asked after immersion. The explanations and justification for the level going up have to be carefully noted, especially as regards the difference between 'it is heavy' and 'it takes up room' (or equivalent expressions).

Items 1, 2 and 3: The same transformations are applied as in the conservation of weight. Before immersion, the psychologist asks: If I put the ball into this glass and the sausage (pancake, all the little bits) into the other, how will the water go up? To the same level in both glasses, or more in one of the glasses? In which one? Can you explain? It is interesting to note whether (with a ball attached to a string) the subject thinks that the level of the water will change according to the degree of immersion (e.g., hanging in the middle of the glass or resting on the bottom).

Item 4: The subject agrees that the ball of clay and the metal ball are identical in size after manipulating them and feeling their weight. The psychologist asks: If I put this ball into one of the glasses and the metal ball into the other, how will the water level be? At the same height, or higher in one of the glasses? In which one? How can you explain that? If the subject gives nonconservation answers, the psychologist actually immerses different objects and notes the eventual effect on the subject's reasoning. An eventual change in reasoning has to be checked on, by a return to one of the traditional items.

Age range: 7 to 12 years.

Task A7. Dissociation between Weight and Volume

Reference: Piaget, J. & Inhelder, B. Le développement des quantités chez l'enfant, chap. XII: 284–325 (Delachaux & Niestlé, 1941 Neuchâtel); translated into English (1974) as: *The child's construction of quantities. Conservation and atomism.* New York: Basic Books.

Materials: 2 identical glasses, 2 rubber bands, 7 cylinders of the same shape and volume; 3 cylinders of aluminum (Aa, Ab, Ac); 1 copper cylinder (Cu); 1 clay cylinder (Pd); 1 cork cylinder (Ck); 1 cylinder made of wax (Wx); 2 aluminum cylinders of the same diameter as Aa, Ab and Ac, but one twice as long (A2) and one three times as long (A3). Each object is attached to a string.

Procedure: The subject agrees that the water goes up to the same level in both glasses (levels are marked with the rubber bands). The psychologist then takes Aa and asks: If I put this cylinder into the water, what will happen? Why do you think the water goes up?

Item 1: The subject is given Aa and Ab to manipulate (same volume, same weight). The psychologist asks: If I put a cylinder into each glass, what is going to happen? How far will the water go up? How would you explain it? After the subject's predictions and justifications, the experimenter immerses the two cylinders (until they rest upright on the bottom of the glasses). The subject is asked: Is that what you thought would happen? In case of a previous nonconservation answer: Why does the water go up to the same level (the same height)?

Item 2: The subject is given Aa and Cu (same volume, different weights). The interview is the same as for item 1 (predictions, explanations, observations of levels after immersion, etc.).

Item 3: The psychologist takes A3 and gives the subject the other cylinder and says: I'm going to put this cylinder into the water in this glass; you figure out what you should put into the other glass so that the level of the water will go up to the same height as in my glass. The psychologist then immerses the A3 cylinder. The subject should first make a choice and explain it, and only then immerse the cylinder(s). The subject then observes what happens, modifies his or her choice or not, and explains.

Item 4: Generalization task. The interview for this item depends on the choice the subject made in item 3. If the subject solved the problem by choosing either A2 plus Ab, or Aa, Ab and Ac (both solutions give the same volume and the same weight), the psychologist proposes that the subject should use different cylinders (e.g., Cu + Ck + A1, or A2 + Cu, A2 + Ck, etc.). The same procedure is used as for item 3.

Item 5: Conservation of volume (only for subjects who solve all the preceding items). The subject is given Aa and the psychologist takes Pd. (a) The psychologist transforms Pd into a long sausage and asks: If I put my sausage into this glass of water so that it is all underneath the water, and you put your cylinder into the other glass, how will the water levels go up? (b) The psychologist transforms Pd into a pancake (cookie) and asks: If I put my cookie into this glass of water and you your cylinder into the other glass, how will the water levels go up? (c) The psychologist transforms Pd into small pieces and asks: If I put all these pieces into this glass of water, and you put your cylinder into the other glass, how will the water levels go up?

Item 6: Effects of the position of the cylinder in the water (provided this problem did not arise during one of the preceding items). The psychologist asks: Do you think the water will go up to the same level or to different levels, when I put one cylinder into the water so that it hangs in the middle, and I let the other one go down so that it rests on the bottom of the other glass?

Note: The psychologist should pay attention to the explanations and remarks of the subject, ask for precision, and invent further items if it is not clear whether the subject argues based on volume or weight, or some other characteristic. For example, if the subject says that Aa and Pd will make the water rise to the same level 'because they are just as big', it is important to know whether the subject means 'high' or 'tall'. The psychologist can then make a clay cylinder of the same height but either thinner or fatter and ask for another prediction.

Age range: 6 to 13 years. This task can also be used with adults, with some modification in the interview.

Task A8. The Dissolution of Sugar: Conservation of Quantity of Matter, Weight, and Volume

Reference: Piaget, J. & Inhelder, B. Le développement des quantités chez l'enfant, chap. IV: 82–98 (Delachaux & Niestlé, 1941 Neuchâtel); translated into English (1974) as: *The child's construction of quantities. Conservation and atomism.* New York: Basic Books.

Materials: 2 identical glasses (same shape, same weight); 2 lumps of sugar; 2 rubber bands; a small stick or spoon; a balance (with two dishes).

Procedure: The psychologist fills the 2 glasses with water (about three-quarters full), puts the rubber bands around the glasses to mark the water level, and places the two glasses on the dishes of the balance, each with a lump of sugar next to it. The subject observes that glass + water + sugar weigh the same.

Part I: Predictions

Item 1: The dissolution of sugar. The psychologist takes the glasses and the sugar lumps from the balance and places them on the table. Several questions are asked: What will happen when I put the sugar lump into this glass of water? What will happen to the sugar and to the water level? Why do you think so; how do you know? How will the water be when the sugar is dissolved? And the sugar? If we let the water evaporate (leaving the glass in the sun for several days), will there be something left at the bottom? What will it look like? If we wait a very long time, will there still be something left? The questions are asked according to the child's responses to preceding questions, and justifications are asked for at several points in the interview.

Item 2: Conservation of quantity of matter. The situation is the same as for item 1. The psychologist asks further questions (and justification after answers): If we make the water evaporate, will we again see the sugar? When the sugar disappears, does it no longer exist? If the sugar is still there, is there still as much as in the lump? If the subject gives nonconservation answers, the psychologist can either ask the weight and volume questions or omit them.

Item 3: Conservation of weight. The psychologist puts the glasses, each with a lump of sugar next to it, on the dishes of the balance. The subject is first asked some questions to make sure that the functioning of the balance is understood: How are the dishes? At the same level? Do you know what that means? Then the subject is asked various questions about the conservation of the weight of the sugar: If we put the sugar into the water and wait till it dissolves, what will happen with the balance? Will the dishes be at the same height? Or will one be higher than the other? Will the glass with the sugar next to it weigh as much as the glass with the dissolved sugar inside it? How do you know? If the subject gives nonconservation answers, the psychologist asks: What should we do to make it the same weight again?

Item 4: Conservation of volume. The situation is the same as in item 3. The psychologist focuses the attention of the subject on the levels of the water: You see, the rubber bands show where the water level is now; in both glasses it is the same height. Do you know what that means? If we put this lump of sugar into this glass, and it dissolves, what will happen to the level of the water? Will it be the same, or higher, or lower? How can you explain? If the subject gives nonconservation answers, the psychologist asks: What should we do so that the levels are again the same?

Part II: Observations

In this part of the task, one of the lumps of sugar is put into the water; dissolution is speeded by stirring. The psychologist waits till the water is again transparent and observes the subject's reaction to the disappearance of the initial opacity. While waiting for the dissolution, the subject is asked to say what s/he expects will happen to the dishes of the balance and to the water levels.

Items 2, 3 and 4 are the same as in Part I. The psychologist asks whether the subject's answers are different from those that were given before, and confronts the subject with eventual discrepancies.

Note. More than in any other Piagetian task, sociocultural and educational factors are important. The task is particularly interesting with subjects who present a certain fragility of mental identity. Their behavior is clearly different from that of educationally or socially disadvantaged subjects.

Age range: 6 to 15 years. The task is also interesting with adults (with appropriate modifications).

Task A9. Conservation and Measurement of Volume

Reference: Piaget, J., Inhelder, B. & Szeminska, A. La géométrie spontanée de l'enfant, chap. IV: 450–478 (Presses Universitaires de France, Paris, 1948); translated into English (1960) as: *The child's conception of geometry.* New York: Basic Books.

Materials: A thick cardboard square, painted blue (38 × 38 cm), representing an expanse of water; 4 pieces of cardboard, 3 × 3 cm (A), 2 × 2 cm (B), 1 × 3 cm (C), and 4 × 3 cm (D), glued to the big cardboard and representing islands; a solid block of wood, 4 cm high on a square base of 3 × 3 cm; 160 small wooden cubes (1 cm). It is often useful to use bigger unit-blocks of 2.5 cm side; the dimensions of the islands are then also multiplied by 2.5 cm.

Procedure: With young children, the psychologist tells a story: The people living on an island (A, 3 × 3 cm solid block) want to move to another island, and want to build a house with just as much room in it as the house they live in now. Just like now, the house will occupy the whole surface of the other island(s). The houses on the other island(s) will be built with the small blocks.

Item 1: The subject is asked to build a house on 2 × 2 cm (B) with the small blocks that has 'just as much room' as the model house (the solid block). The psychologist asks first what the subject thinks the house will look like, and then lets the subject take as long as necessary to finish the construction. Some young subjects may need help in keeping the blocks correctly aligned. The psychologist then asks: How did you do it? Is there just as much room as in the old house? Are the two houses just as big, with just as much room? How can you be sure? What would you do to make sure that it is the same? The psychologist can refer to real situations: Why do architects build skyscrapers; do they need less ground? If there is not much space, and a lot of people are to live in a building, what does one do? The subject is allowed to manipulate the solid block, but if s/he proposes to make a copy of it using the small blocks, the psychologist says that that will be done later. (It is a useful additional item after the task is finished in its traditional form.) The subject's construction is left as it is.

Item 2: The subject is asked to build another house on 1 × 3 cm (C) with just as much room on another island. The technique is the same as for item 1.

Item 3: The subject is asked to build yet another house on 4 × 3 cm (D) on a third island. The technique is the same as for items 1 and 2.

Item 4: Transitivity. The four houses remain present, and questions such as the following are asked: Does this house (B) have just as much room as this one (C)? And these other two (B and D)? Similarly, house D will be compared to B and C. Justifications and explanations are requested.

Item 5: Proportions. Questions are asked such as the following: Can you tell me how much higher (or lower) this house (B, C or D) is than the model house (A)?

Notes: (1) The psychologist should carefully note the way the subject goes about the construction, and sometimes ask questions, without, however, interrupting too often. Only when the subject seems to be extremely dependent on the adult should the psychologist respond to the subject's appeals for help; all such appeals and the actual help given should precisely be noted.

(2) This task also relates to category D below.

(3) This task is particularly interesting for the analysis of relational and interactional behavior. If the subject is not greatly inhibited, it is an ideal task for the beginning of a psychological investigation. It provides the psychologist with insight into the subject's planning capacities and level of mental autonomy.

Age range: 5 to 14–15 years. With modification, the task is also interesting with adults.

Task A10. Drawing Episodes of Activities during One Day

Reference: Task used by the late A. Jaeggi in the Service Médico-pédagogique in Geneva. No bibliographical reference has been found.

Materials: A sheet of paper folded in sixths; a blue pencil.

Procedure: The psychologist unfolds the paper and says: I want you to draw a little story for me. There's a boy or girl who has a whole day free to do what s/he likes. Make me a drawing of what s/he is going to do from when s/he gets up in the morning and comes out of his/her house (the first rectangle is indicated as being at the top left) until s/he comes back home in the evening (rectangle 6, bottom right). The subject is left to make the drawings without interruption. When the strip is finished, the subject is asked to tell the story for which the drawings were made. The narration should be noted precisely.

Note: This task is particularly informative as regards the evaluation of the permanence of the subject's psychical identity through the analysis of the procedures used, the affects and judgements, the relational and social behaviors and the internal reference points of the identificatory movements.

Age range: 4 years and above.

Category B
Symbolic Constructions [Schmid-Kitsikis et al., 1987]

Only one task will be described in this category. This task is in the experimental stage and has not as yet been standardized. Other tasks are used in this category, such as free drawing or drawings as in task A10. The task described (B1) is particularly informative as regards the subject's symbolic activities (both public and private) and allows the psychologist to observe how the subject integrates primary and secondary processes. In this last aspect the task is closely related to category D.

Task B1. Symbolic Activity and Creativity

Materials: 24 small objects (dolls, toy animals and miniature objects used in daily life): a man, a woman, a baby; a crocodile and a wolf-hound or a rabbit (made of plastic); a teddy-bear, a dolphin and a soft furry rabbit; a pot with lid, a knife, a fork, a bowl; a mirror, a comb, a toilet; a dog kennel; a carrot, a loaf of bread, a babybottle (with milk that seems to vanish when the bottle is inclined); a spanner, pincers, scissors; modelling clay and a square of soft woolly material.

Procedure: Psychologist and subject are seated next to one another at a table (suitable for the subject), on which materials are placed randomly.

Item 1: Spontaneous phase. The psychologist says, pointing to the objects: Do you see all these things? You can do with them what you like and say what you like, too. If the subject remains inactive and silent, the psychologist waits for about a minute (less, if the subject shows anxiety and simply touches or displaces the objects). If the subject still remains inactive or if s/he only classifies the objects, the psychologist suggests: Can you play a story for me? This phase of the task lasts about 30 min.

Item 2: Directed phase. With the same objects on the table, again arranged randomly, the psychologist asks: Do you see all these things? Do you think you could put them in some order? After the subject has made a first arrangement, the psychologist asks for a description or explanation, then suggests: Could you put together all those that go together? If the subject has difficulties, s/he is told that for easier isolation of a group, s/he can ask for a piece of paper whenever s/he has an idea of what to put together ...

'as many pieces of paper you need, but try to use as few as possible'. If the subject cannot sort the objects or cannot change the criterion for sorting, the psychologist suggests 4 groupings by putting on 4 pieces of paper a person (the man), an animal (the dog), a tool (spanner), a food (bread), and asks the subject to continue.

Notes: (1) All activities, attitudes, remarks and expressions should be noted, as well as the subject's descriptions of the grouping and configurations into which the objects are put. If the subject spontaneously includes some other objects, or makes up an object, this should also be noted, as well as marked changes in the tempo of actions.

(2) This task is also useful in the analysis of the subject's psychological identity (category A).

Age range: 3 to 12 years.

Category C
Construction of Images (Graphic Representations)

Task C1. Translation of a Square Relative to Another Square

Reference: Piaget, J. & Inhelder, B. L'image mentale chez l'enfant, chap. III: 64–67 (Presses Universitaires de France, Paris, 1966); translated into English (1971) as: *Mental imagery in the child. A study of the development of imaginal representation.* New York: Basic Books.

Materials: 2 pieces of blue cardboard, 5 cm square (A and B); 2 pieces of blue cardboard, 5 cm square (A′ and B′) with a 1 cm long red line drawn on each at right angles from the middle of one side; 2 pieces of blue cardboard, 5 cm square (A″ and B″), with 1 cm long lines drawn on each, 1 cm from the corner at right angles to one side; paper and pencil; a series of prepared drawings, showing the correct solution and some frequently observed mistakes.

Procedure: The psychologist takes the 2 pieces of cardboard without lines and places them one above the other, so that they touch along the whole of one side. The psychologist first asks the subject to draw this configuration.

Item 1: (a) The subject is asked to draw the situation that will result when square A is moved slightly to the right, with square B remaining immobile. (The psychologist makes a small movement with his or her finger indicating a lateral displacement to the right of about 1 cm.) The subject is asked: Can you guess what the squares will look like and make a drawing? The instruction is repeated as often as is necessary for the subject to understand it, but the square is not actually displaced. (b) Using the same two squares, the psychologist asks: And now can you draw what the squares will look like if I push this one (A) a bit further (indicating a displacement to the right of about 2.5 cm)? (c) The psychologist asks: And what will the squares look like if I push this one (A) even further (movement with finger to beyond square B)?

Item 2: As in item 1, but with simultaneous displacements. The psychologist places his or her right index finger on A, left on B, and sketches movements to left and right (without actually displacing the squares).

Item 3: (a) The psychologist takes squares A′ and B′ and presents them one above the other, with the 2 red lines aligned and contiguous. The interview proceeds as in item 1.

(b) The psychologist takes squares A″ and B″ and again presents them one above the other, but this time with the red lines at the left of the upper and right of the lower square. The psychologist asks: When I push this square (A″) until its line touches the line of this one (B″), can you make a drawing of what the squares will look like?

Item 4: The series of drawings is presented to those subjects who have difficulties. The subject is asked to choose the drawings that correspond to Item Ia, Ib and Ic.

Age range: 4 to 8 years.

Task C2. Rotation of a Square Relative to Another Square

Reference: Piaget, J. & Inhelder, B. L'image mentale chez l'enfant, chap. IV: 132–141 (Presses Universitaires de France, Paris, 1966); translated into English (1971) as: *Mental imagery in the child. A study of the development of imaginal representation.* New York: Basic Books.

Materials: A piece of thick cardboard (30 cm square); a piece of blue cardboard (5 cm square) glued to the middle of the thick cardboard; a piece of red cardboard (5 cm square) nailed at its corner to a corner of the blue square, so that it can rotate to a position superimposed over the blue square; a series of prepared drawings, showing correct solutions and some frequently observed mistakes.

Procedure: The psychologist shows the material to the subject and demonstrates that the blue square is glued onto the cardboard, but that the red square can be made to turn, with the nail as a pivot.

Item 1: Anticipation. The subject is asked to imagine and to draw the positions of the red square in relation to the blue square when it is pushed little by little. At least 8 different positions, including a 360 degrees rotation, should be asked for; at most 16. For each new drawing, the immediately preceding drawing is kept in view; the earlier drawings are taken away. If the subject only draws rotations of 90, 180, 270 and 360 degrees, the psychologist should ask for intermediate positions. At no point in the interview is the red square actually rotated. The psychologist should ask for drawings that show the position of the nail.

Item 2: Recognition. The series of drawings is presented and the subject has to choose drawings that represent positions the red square can actually occupy during a 360 degree rotation.

Item 3: Copy. For the subject who has difficulties in imagining the various positions of the red square in relation to the blue one, the psychologist actually rotates the square into various positions and asks the subject to draw the configuration as shown. This task makes it possible to decide whether erroneous anticipatory drawings were due to graphic difficulties or not. Item 1 can be repeated following item 3. Modifications in the drawings are noted and can be commented upon.

Age range: 6 to 10 years.

Task C3. The Projection of Shadows

Reference: Piaget, J. & Inhelder, B. La représentation de l'espace chez l'enfant, chap. VII: 231–242 (Presses Universitaires de France, Paris, 1948); translated into English (1956) as: *The child's conception of space.* Atlantic Highlands: The Humanities Press.

Materials: A white screen (40 cm square) placed vertically on a support; a candle in a candlestick; a thin metal stick (10 cm long, cross-section 2 mm); a metal ring (10 cm in diameter, cross-section 2 mm); pincers to hold the stick and the ring; a series of drawings of various shadows projected by stick and ring, including correct solutions as well as frequently observed mistakes; paper and pencil.

Procedure: The subject is seated in the axis of the projection, facing the screen with the candle between. No shadow should be visible as long as the candle is not lit.

Item 1: Understanding what causes shadows. The psychologist explores the subject's ideas about shadows. After lighting the candle and showing briefly the shadow produced by an object (different from those used in the following item), the subject is asked: What does one see on the screen? What does it mean? Why is there a shadow? When does one see shadows? If I took a transparent object, would there be a shadow?

Item 2: Positions of the stick. The candle is extinguished, and the psychologist holds the metal stick vertically between the candle and the screen. The subject is asked 'to draw the shadow of the stick as it will be on the screen when the candle is lit'. Then the psychologist tilts the stick first 30 degrees, then 60 degrees (top part toward the subject) and asks for another drawing. Finally the stick is held horizontally, pointing to the screen, and a drawing is asked for.

Item 3: Positions of the ring. The same positions are presented as in item 2, but with the ring. After the subject has made drawings for these two items, the psychologist asks for explanations, e.g., why some drawings do not look like rings or sticks (or why they do, if the subject has drawn them thus).

Item 4: Choice of drawings. For those subjects who had difficulties with items 2 and 3, the psychologist presents the series of drawings, first those of the stick in its various positions, then those of the ring (the drawings are presented in random order). Items 2 and 3 are then repeated, and the subject is asked to choose the drawings that correspond to the positions.

Item 5: Drawing of the shadows as they appear on the screen with the candle lit. The same positions as in items 2 and 3 are presented and the subject is asked to make a drawing of their shadows. The psychologist should note differences between the drawings made for item 2 and 3 and those made when the candle is actually lit.

Note: This task is also interesting for analysis of the psychological identity of the subject; it should be related to the subject's responses to tasks in category A.

Age range: 7 to 14–15 years.

Category D
Logical Reasoning: Logico-Mathematical Constructions

Task D1. Seriation by Length

Reference: Piaget, J. & Szeminska, A. La genèse du nombre chez l'enfant, chap. IX: 251–262 (Delachaux & Niestlé, 1941 Neuchâtel); translated into English (1952) as: *The child's conception of number.* Atlantic Highlands: The Humanities Press.

Materials: A series of 10 small sticks ranging from 16 to 10.6 cm in length, each differing in length from the next by 0.6 cm; the same series of 10 sticks glued parallel onto a piece of cardboard, each 1.5 cm distant from the next with their bases aligned; 10 small sticks ranging from 15.7 to 10.3 cm in length; a screen (30 × 50 cm).

Procedure: The subject is given the first series of sticks in a pile.

Item 1: Seriation without a screen. The psychologist says: I would like you to put these sticks in order, one next to the other flat on the table, so that they make a kind of staircase; can you tell me how you are going to do it? If necessary, the psychologist can demonstrate what is wanted by arranging the first two sticks in the right ascending order and asking the subject to continue. The psychologist notes how the subject selects each stick, the order in which they are arranged, and the shape of the 'staircase'. If the subject makes a more or less correct ascending line as regards the tops of the sticks, but without keeping their bases aligned, the psychologist asks for 'a prettier staircase' and may give some help with the first sticks. After the subject has finished, the psychologist says: Tell me how you chose the sticks.

Item 2: Insertion of the third series into the series glued onto the cardboard. The subject is given the cardboard with the sticks glued onto it, and the psychologist hands him or her the sticks of the third series in the following order (1 = the longest stick): 3, 9, 1, 8, 5, 10, 6, 4, 7, 2. With each stick the psychologist asks: If you have to fit this stick in with the others that are already glued down, where should it go? The subject's strategies are observed and recorded.

Item 3: Seriation behind a screen. The subject is seated with the screen between subject and psychologist. The psychologist says: This time, I am going to put down the sticks so that they are in order, making a good staircase; you give them to me one by one, in the right order for the staircase. The psychologist should not let the subject construct the seriation on the table before handing the stick over. If the subject makes a mistake, the screen is lifted so that the already placed sticks are visible and the order can be rectified. When the subject has given the psychologist 5 or 6 sticks, s/he is asked: How long is the next one? (suggesting a comparison both with the sticks that are already placed behind the screen and with those that are still to be placed).

Note: This task is interesting for the analysis of the subject's planning capacities.

Age range: 4 to 8 years.

Task D2. Sorting Task with Varying Criteria

Reference: Piaget, J. & Inhelder, B. La genèse des structures logiques élémentaires, chap. VII: 210–218 and Chap. VI: 168–178 (Delachaux & Niestlé, 1959 Neuchâtel); translated into English (1964) as: *The early growth of logic in the child. Classification and seriation.* London: Harper and Row.

Materials: (a) Geometrical shapes cut from cardboard: 2 red and 2 blue circles, diameter 25 mm; 2 red and 2 blue circles, diameter 50 mm; 2 red and 2 blue 25 mm squares; 2 red and 2 blue 50 mm squares. (b) Drawings of persons on 8 × 8 cm cards (one person per card): 4 men: a policeman, a clown, a footballer, a man in evening dress; 4 women: one with a hat, one with a basket, one with a pail, one on skis; 4 boys: one with a satchel, one with a shopping bag, one running, one playing with a football; 4 girls: one with a handbag, one running, one with a dog, one with a doll. (c) Drawings of vehicles on 8 × 8 cm cards: 8 vehicles with and without a motor, two-wheeled or four-wheeled (e.g., a car, a truck, a baby carriage, a supermarket trolley, a motorcycle, a motor-scooter, a bicycle, a child's scooter).

Procedure: All the objects are put in a heap on the table in the order described and the subject is asked to describe them: Tell me what's there.

Item 1: Spontaneous sorting. The psychologist asks the subject: Can you put together all those that go together? When the subject has finished, the psychologist asks: Why did you put all these together? And all those? What would you call this lot? And that? If the subject spontaneously divides the objects into two groups, item 2 is skipped.

Item 2: Dichotomization. The subject is asked: Now could you put them all into just two piles? Could you put one pile on this sheet of paper and the other one on that one? When the subject is finished, the psychologist asks: Why did you put all these together? What could you call this pile? If the subject has difficulty in finding a description for the grouping, s/he is asked to name some of the objects; the psychologist can also insert an inappropriate object into one of the piles and ask: If I put this one here, would that be okay? Why? Why not?

Item 3: First change of criterion. The psychologist mixes the objects again and asks the subject: Could you arrange them any other way in two piles? If the subject repeats the first solution, the psychologist says: You've already done it like that; can you find a different way of putting them together in two piles? If necessary, the psychologist initiates a new method of sorting and asks the subject to continue. The interview continues as in item 2.

Item 4: Second change of criterion. The psychologist asks: Can you find yet another way of putting them in two piles? The interview continues as in items 2 and 3.

Notes: (1) It is often interesting to ask for the subject's ideas before the actual sorting starts: Can you tell me before you start how you are going to do it? What are you going to put together? Why?

(2) It is interesting to use at least materials (a) *and* (b), or (a) *and* (c) and to note possible differences in the subject's strategies.

Age range: 3 to 10 years.

Task D3. Quantification of Class Inclusion

Reference: Inhelder, B., Sinclair, H. & Bovet, M. Apprentissage et structures de la connaissance, chap. VII: 205–231 (Presses Universitaires de France, Paris, 1974); translated into English (1974) as: *Learning and the development of cognition.* Cambridge, Mass.: Harvard University Press.

Materials: 12 oranges (plastic miniatures are used for all the fruit) (O); 12 apples (A); 2 lemons (L); 2 pears (P); 1 banana (B); 2 dolls, a girl and a boy; 2 baskets.

Procedure: The psychologist asks the subject to name the fruit and to make sure the generic term 'fruit' or 'piece of fruit' is known. This task raises problems in the English version; in French, there is a singular *un fruit* and a plural *des fruits,* but in English 'fruit' is normally a collective noun and 'fruits' refers to different kinds of fruit. In the description, 'pieces of fruit' will be used for the French plural *fruits;* it may, however, be better, for English-speaking subjects, to avoid the problem by replacing the fruit by different kinds of cookies or candies. The two dolls, each with a basket, are put on the table.

Item 1: Two collections. The psychologist puts these items into one of the baskets: OOOOAA. The subject is asked: Put into the other basket more apples, because the girl likes apples better, but just as many pieces of fruit, so that it is fair, so that nobody is jealous.

Variations: (1) The psychologist puts into one of the baskets AAOOLL and tells the subject to put into the other doll's basket 'more oranges, but just as many pieces of fruit (the same number)'. (2) The psychologist puts into one basket AAAOPB and tells the subject to put into the other one 'just as many pieces of fruit, but fewer apples'.

Item 2: Only one basket remains on the table. The psychologist puts into it AAAAAOPL and asks: Are there more apples or more pieces of fruit? How do you know? Can you explain? Then OOOPPP are placed in the basket, and the following questions are asked: Are there more pieces of fruit or more oranges, or just as many pieces of fruit as oranges? How do you know? Can you explain? Finally the psychologist places into the basket PPPPPPPP and asks: Are there more apples than pieces of fruit, or just as many? How do you know? Can you explain?

Age range: 5 to 10 years.

Task D4. Classification of Animals

Reference: Piaget, J. & Inhelder, B. La genèse des structures logiques élémentaires, chap. IV: 113–122 (Delachaux & Niestlé, 1959); translated into English (1964) as: *The early growth of logic in the child. Classification and seriation.* London: Harper and Row.

Materials: 25 cards (6 × 6 cm square) containing drawings of: 5 poodles (A); 5 dogs other than poodles (B); 5 animals other than dogs (C); a book; a tree; 3 transparent envelopes of different sizes; 3 labels on which the words 'poodles', 'dogs', and 'animals' are written.

Procedure: The psychologist first asks the subject to name all the animals and objects drawn on the cards.

Item 1: (a) Spontaneous sorting. The subject is asked: Can you put together the pictures that go together? Make some piles of those that resemble one another. When the subject has finished, the psychologist asks for a description of the piles the subject has made. (b) Suggested sorting. The subject is asked: Can you make 3 piles? If the subject does so, the psychologist asks for a name for each pile. If the subject has difficulties, the psychologist starts 3 piles with 1 or 2 elements, and, if necessary, completes the sorting. The subject is then given the 3 envelopes and the psychologist suggests putting pile A into the smallest, pile B into the next largest, and pile C into the largest envelope. The subject is asked whether this seems a good way of sorting and why. The labels with the names can be put on the envelopes.

Item 2: (a) Hierarchical classification. The psychologist asks: Can we put this envelope (poodles) into this one (dogs)? And call them together 'dogs'? Can you explain? The psychologist then takes one of the non-poodle dogs and starts to put it into the poodle envelope and asks: Would it also be okay if I put this picture in with the poodles and still kept the same label (poodles)? Why? Why not? Similar questions are then asked about the pictures of dogs and animals other than dogs. (b) Subtraction of classes. The psychologist asks: If someone took away all the poodles in the world, would there be any dogs left? If someone took away all the dogs, would there be any poodles left? If someone took away all the animals, would there be any dogs left? After each response the psychologist asks for justifications. (c) Quantification of class inclusion. The psychologist takes 4 pictures of poodles and 3 of other dogs and asks: Are there more poodles or more dogs? The psychologist takes 4 pictures of dogs and 3 pictures of other animals and asks: Are there more animals or more dogs? And in the whole world, are there more animals or more dogs? After each response, the subject is asked for justifications.

Age range: 6 to 12 years.

Task D5. Combination of Operations

Reference: Piaget, J. & Inhelder, B. La genèse de l'idée de hasard chez l'enfant, chap. IX: 208–225 (Presses Universitaires de France, Paris, 1951); translated into English (1975) as: *The origin of the idea of chance in children.* Henley-on-Thames: Routledge and Kegan.

Materials: 5 decks of 30 cards each (2 × 2 cm), one deck with all the cards marked with the number 1, one deck with 2, one deck with 3, one deck with 4, and one deck with 5.

Procedure: The psychologist first explores the subject's knowledge of two-digit numbers: Do you know any numbers you write with two numerals (numbers, digits)? How far can you count? How do you write fifteen?

Item 1: The subject is given the decks of cards marked 1 and 2. The psychologist asks: How many different numbers of two digits can you make with these? The subject is then asked to actually make the numbers with cards: Make as many different numbers as you can with ones and twos. If the subject only produces 2 numbers, the psychologist may help: Look, you can also make these. After the subject has finished, the psychologist asks: How did you work it out? How do you know that is all? How do you know you did not do the same one twice? If the subject has not arranged the numbers systematically, the psychologist helps the subject to do so.

Item 2: The psychologist adds deck 3. The interview proceeds as for item 1. The psychologist makes it clear that two-digit numbers are to be constructed.

Items 3 and 4: The subject is given the other decks and the same questions are asked. No exhaustive arrangements are requested, only verbal answers.

Item 5: The psychologist asks for a recapitulation of what has been found out with the preceding items, and then asks: Is there some kind of a rule to know quickly how many different two-digit numbers can be made up with even more cards, say also cards that are marked 6, 7, or even more?

Age range: 6 to 14 years.

Task D6. Quantification of Probabilities

Reference: Piaget, J. & Inhelder, B. La genèse de l'idée de hasard chez l'enfant, chap. VI: 144–173 (Presses Universitaires de France, Paris, 1951); translated into English (1975) as: *The origin of the idea of chance in children.* Henley-on-Thames: Routledge and Kegan.

Materials: 25 white counters, 10 marked with a cross on one side.

Procedure: The subject is asked to put the counters into 2 piles, those with a cross and those without. The psychologist then says: Now look carefully, I'm going to put some counters together here, and some others there, and then I will turn the ones with a cross over, so that they all look alike; you will have to remember where the crosses are.

For each of the following *12 items,* the psychologist then puts down 2 differently composed collections of counters, A and B. (The numerator indicates the number of crosses, the denominator the total number of counters in the collection.)

Item	Collection A	Collection B
1	1/2	2/2
2	1/2	0/2
3	2/3	2/3
4	2/5	1/5
5	1/3	1/2
6	2/4	3/4
7	2/5	2/3
8	1/2	2/4
9	1/2	2/5
10	2/3	3/5
11	1/3	2/6
12	2/5	3/7

Starting with the first item (unless the subject appears too advanced for this simple situation), the psychologist asks: If you could only make one draw, take one counter from either this pile or that one, in which pile would you have the best chance of getting a counter with a cross? Why? How do you know? The subject is then allowed to turn over the crosses of each collection, and the psychologist may ask the subject to count the crosses and the total number of counters in each collection. The counters with crosses are then once again turned over, or, for subjects who have great difficulties, covered by the psychologist.

Age range: 7 years and above.

Task D7. Isolation of Variables

Reference: Inhelder, B. & Piaget, J. De la logique de l'enfant à la logique de l'adolescent, chap. VII: 97–110 (Presses Universitaires de France, Paris, 1955); translated into English (1958) as: *The growth of logical thinking from childhood to adolescence. An essay on the construction of formal operational structures.* New York: Basic Books. (This task is a modification of the task described in the reference; the underlying principles are the same but different material is used.)

Materials: A switchboard with an electric bulb and 5 sockets into which 5 plugs (A, B, C, D and E) can be inserted. The plugs are identical in appearance and their wiring to the switchboard is not easily discernible. The 5 plugs work as follows: When A, C and D are inserted, the bulb is turned on; when B is inserted, the bulb is turned off; E has no effect.

Procedure: The psychologist shows the subject the lamp. The subject is given the 5 plugs and shown that they fit into the 5 sockets on the switchboard.

Item 1: The psychologist says: Try to light the lamp. You can use any or all of the plugs, but try to find out quickly; think about what you do, and don't make too many useless tries. The psychologist notes all the actions and remarks of the subject. When the subject isolates the correct combination (using plugs A, C, and D) for lighting the lamp, the psychologist asks whether there would be yet another combination that would give the same effect, and how the subject would explain the system to somebody else. The subject is then asked to explain the respective effects of the combination ACD (the only effective combination to light the lamp), of B (which extinguishes the light) and of E (which has no effect at all).

Item 2: For subjects who cannot manage to find the combination that lights the lamp nor the effects of plugs B and E, the psychologist offers help, by showing what happens when ACD are plugged in, and what the effects of B and E are. Once the subject has learned this, s/he is asked to prove (a) that E has no effect, (b) that B extinguishes the lamp once it is lit, and (c) that forgetting to plug in one of the plugs ACD does not have the same effect as plugging in B. With subjects who did not spontaneously solve the problem but understood it during item 2, the psychologist then asks for a recapitulation of the effects produced by the various plugs. (The subject is allowed to use pencil and paper.) All manipulations and remarks, as well as request for help, are noted in detail.

Note: This task yields information on the relational and interactional characteristics of the subject and on the subject's mental and psychological autonomy.

Age range: 6 years and above.

Task D8. Rey's Complex Figure

Reference: Rey, A. Test de la figure complexe (Editions du Centre de Psychologie Appliquée, Paris, 1959).

The task consists in copying and then reproducing from memory a complex line figure. The figure combines the following characteristics:

- there is no obvious meaning,
- it does not call for draughtsmanship,
- it is sufficiently complicated to call for perceptive, analytical and organizational activity.

Task D9. Kohs-Goldstein's Test, as Adapted by R. Zazzo

Reference: Zazzo, R. Manuel pour l'examen psychologique de l'enfant (Delachaux & Niestlé, 1969).

This task presents a series of mosaic models that are to be reproduced with a certain number of cubes. The models are arranged in increasing order of difficulty.

The task serves to analyze the type and degree of difficulty of 'abstractive behaviors', abstraction permitting space to be analyzed and structured.

Appendix B

Assessment Summary

The following outline is useful in summarizing the psychological assessment of a child.

I. Behavior

To be described in detail plus its development during the sessions.

1. Motoric.
2. Expressive.
3. Relational.

II. Acquisitions

According to levels or periods of acquisition; establishment of a profile.

1. Language (vocabulary, grammar, structure of discourse, phonatory quality, communicative value, etc.).
2. Motricity (corporal, manual, lateralization).
3. Intellectual acquisitions (according to criteria used in scales of intellectual development).
4. Physical and numerical invariants (concepts of conservation).
5. Logic of classes and relations.
6. Space (topological, projective, Euclidian).
7. Imagery, mental images (reproduction, evocation).
8. Memory (short- and long-term).
9. Conventional symbolization (play, drawing).
10. School achievement (reading, writing, spelling, arithmetic).
11. Rules and social conduct.

III. Mental and Relational Functioning

1. Emotions and affects (modes of expression or repression, degree of differentiation, movement and/or modification of affects). Relations: affects/reality; affects/internal states (corporal movements, sensations of pleasure/displeasure).
2. Modes of interaction (with objects and persons, in the start and pursuit of an exchange).

3A. Object relations (choice and cathexis of objects according to their type – total, partial, phantasmic, animated/inanimate; degree of differentiation between internal and external objects and their qualities; value of a symptom; secondary benefits).
3B. Modes of object relations between partners – development and deviance (analysis of mechanisms – splitting of the ego and of the object, incorporation/excorporation, introjection/projection, assimilation/accommodation, denial/idealization).
4A. Identity (narcissistic and parental imagos and their degree of differentiation; systems of sexual and social identification and their importance for ego organization).
4B. Developmental and defensive value of representations.
4C. State of the id, ego, superego, ideal ego.
5. Fantasy (thematic organization, level of picturability, type and process of elaboration, links with affects and reality).
6. Thought (mobility, autonomy, creativity, developmental and regressive movements; private symbolic thought and conventional symbolic thought).

IV. Psychological Diagnosis

Cathexes, acquisitions, organizations, functioning and mental development.

V. Psychological Prognosis

Probable development of mental and environmental conditions; recommended treatment; possibilities of adjustment.

References

Anzieu, D. (1985). *Le psychodrame analytique chez l'enfant.* Paris: Presses Universitaires de France.

Apostel, L. (1959). *Logique et apprentissage. Etudes d'épistémologie génétique.* Paris: Presses Universitaires de France.

Basquin, M., Dubuisson, P., Samuel-Lajeunesse, B., & Testemale-Monod, G. (1972). *Le psychodrame: Une approche psychanalytique.* Paris: Dunod.

Bates, E. (1979). *The emergence of symbols.* New York: Academic Press.

Bégoin-Guignard, F. (1985a). Limites et lieux de la psychose et de l'interprétation. *Topique, 35/36,* 173–184.

Bégoin-Guignard, F. (1985b). Ballade au préconscient: Les pulsions et leurs objets et la relation «contenant-contenu». *Revue Française de Psychanalyse, 5,* 1391–1400.

Bégoin-Guignard, F. (1988). Object et réalité: Esquisse sur le connu et l'inconnu de l'objet. *Topique, 42,* 207–222.

Bion, W.R. (1962). *Learning from experience.* New York: Basic Books.

Bion, W.R. (1963). *Elements of psychoanalysis.* London: Heinemann.

Bion, W.R. (1965). *Transformations: Change from learning to growth.* London: Heinemann.

Bion W.R. (1967). *Second thoughts.* London: Heinemann.

Brauschweig, D., & Fain, M. (1975). *La nuit et le jour: Essai psychanalytique sur le fonctionnement mental.* Paris: Presses Universitaires de France.

Cooper, L.A., & Shepard, R.N. (1973). Chronometric studies of the rotation of mental images. In W.G. Chase (Ed.), *Visual information processing.* New York: Academic Press.

Denis, M. (1979). *Les images mentales.* Paris: Presses Universitaires de France.

Dick, A.O. (1974). Iconic memory and its relation to perceptual processing and other memory mechanisms. *Perception and Psychophysics, 16,* 575–596.

Euse, F.J., & Haney, J.N. (1975). Clarity, controllability, and emotional intensity of image: Correlations with introversion, neuroticism and subjective anxiety. *Perceptual and Motor Skills, 40,* 443–447.

Fain, M., & Dejours, C. (1974). *Corps malade et corps érotique.* Paris: Masson.

Fedida, P. (1968). Perception et compréhension clinique en psychologie. *Bulletin de Psychologie No Spécial T. XXI, 270,* 908–929.

Freud, S. (1900). *Die Traumdeutung.* Vienna G.S., II–III; G.W. II–III.

Furth, H.G. (1966). *Thinking without language: Psychological implications of deafness.* New York: Free Press.

Furth, H.G. (1971). Linguistic deficiency and thinking: Research with deaf subjects 1964–1969. *Psychological Bulletin, 76,* 58–72.

Gibeault, A. (1982). Symbolisme primitif et formation des symboles. «L'archaïque», *Nouvelle Revue de Psychanalyse, 26,* 293–321.

Green, A. (1987). La capacité de rêverie et le mythe étiologique. *Revue Française de Psychanalyse LI, Juillet–Septembre,* 1299–1317.

Hoffmann, J., Denis, M., & Ziessler, M. (1983). Figurative features and the construction of visual images. *Psychological Research, 45,* 39–54.

Holt, R.R. (1964). Imagery: The return of the ostracized. *American Psychologist, 19,* 254–264.

Horowitz, M.J. (1976). *Image formation and cognition.* New York: Appleton-Century-Craft.

Huckabee, M.W. (1974). Introversion-extraversion and imagery. *Psychological Reports, 34,* 453–454.

Inhelder, B., Lézine, I., Sinclair, H., & Stambak, M. (1972). Les débuts de la fonction symbolique. *Archives de Psychologie XLI, 163,* 187–243.

Kamii, C., & Devries, R. (1978). *Physical knowledge in preschool education: Implications of Piaget's theory.* Englewood Clifts NJ: Prentice-Hall.

Klein, M. (1930). *Die Bedeutung der Symbolbildung für die Ichentwicklung.* I.Z.P; translated into English (1930) as: *The importance of symbolformation for the development of the Ego;* in (1948) Contributions to Psycho-Analysis. London: Hogarth Press.

Klein, M. (1932). *The psychoanalysis of children.* London: Hogarth Press.

Klein, M. (1940). *Mourning and its relation to manic-depression States;* in (1948) Contributions to Psycho-Analysis. London: Hogarth Press.

Klein, M. (1952). *Some theoretical conclusions regarding the emotional life of the infant;* in Develop. in Psychoanal. London: Hogarth Press.

Kreisler, L., Fain, M., & Soulé, M. (1984). *L'enfant et son corps.* Paris: Presses Universitaires de France.

Mahler, M.S. (1968). *Infantile psychosis.* New York: International Universities Press.

Mahler, M.S., Pine, F., & Bergman, A. (1975). *The psychological birth of the human infant.* New York: Basic Books.

Marty, P. (1976). *Les mouvements individuels de vie et de mort.* Paris: Payot.

Marty, P. (1980). *L'ordre psychosomatique.* Paris: Payot.

Marty, P., de M'Uzan, M., & David, C. (1963). *L'investigation psychosomatique.* Paris: Presses Universitaires de France.

Meltzer, D. (1972). *Sexual states of mind.* Perth: Clunie Press.

Meltzer, D. (1975). *Explorations in autism: A psychoanalytical study.* Perth: Clunie Press.

Meltzer, D. (1978). *The Kleinian development.* The Rolan Harris Educational Trust. Perth: Clunie Press.

Meyerson, I. (1932). Les images. In G. Dumas (Ed.), *Nouveau traité de psychologie, tome II: Les fondements de la vie mentale.* Paris: Alcan.

de M'Uzan, M. (1977). *De l'art à la mort.* Paris: Gallimard.

Neisser, U. (1972). Changing conceptions of imagery. In P.W. Sheehan (Ed.), *The function and nature of imagery.* New York: Academic Press.

Orsini-Bouichou, F. (1982). *L'intelligence de l'enfant, ontogenèse des invariants.* Paris: Editions C.N.R.S.

Orsini-Bouichou, F., & Paour, J.-L. (1986). Cognitive change and behaviour. In P.L.C. van Geert (Ed.), *Theory building in developmental psychology.* Amsterdam: North-Holland.

Paivio, A. (1969). Mental imagery in associative learning and memory. *Psychol. Rev., 76,* 241–263.
Paivio, A. (1977). Images, propositions and knowledge. In S.M. Nicholas (Ed.), *Images, perception and knowledge.* Dordrecht: Reidel.
Paour, J.-L. (1979). Apprentissage des notions de conservation et induction de la pensée opératoire concrète chez les débiles mentaux. In R. Zazzo (Ed.), *Les débilités mentales.* Paris: Armand Colin.
Paour, J.-L. (1985). De l'induction des structures logiques à la modification du fonctionnement cognitif chez les retardés intellectuels. *Revue Suisse de Psychologie, 44,* 135–147.
Paour, J.L. (1987). Retard mental et aides cognitives. In S.P. Caverni, C. Bastien, P. Mendelsohn & G. Tiberghien (Eds.), *Psychologie cognitive: modèles et méthodes.* Grenoble: Presses Universitaires de Grenoble.
Perron, R. (1985). *Genèse de la personne.* Paris: Presses Universitaires de France.
Piaget, J. (1936). *La naissance de l'intelligence chez l'enfant.* Neuchâtel: Delachaux & Niestlé; translated into English (1952) as: *The origins of intelligence in children.* New York: International Universities Press.
Piaget, J. (1937). *La construction du réel chez l'enfant.* Neuchâtel: Delachaux & Niestlé; translated into English (1954) as: *The construction of reality in the child.* New York: Basic Books.
Piaget, J. (1945). *La formation du symbole chez l'enfant.* Neuchâtel: Delachaux & Niestlé; translated into English (1951) as: *Play dreams and imitation in childhood.* New York: Norton.
Piaget, J., & Inhelder, B (1966). *L'image mentale chez l'enfant.* Paris: Presses Universitaires de France; translated into English (1971) as: *Mental imagery in the child. A study of the development of imaginal representation.* New York: Basic Books.
Piaget, J. (1967a). *Biologie et connaissance.* Paris: Gallimard; translated into English (1971) as: *Biology and knowledge. An essay on the relation between organic regulations and cognitive processes.* Chicago: University of Chicago Press.
Piaget, J., et al. (1967b). *Logique et connaissance scientifique.* Paris: Gallimard.
Piaget, J. (1968a). *Mémoire et intelligence.* Paris: Presses Universitaives de France; translated into English (1973) as: *Memory and intelligence.* New York: Basic Books.
Piaget, J., Sinclair, H., & Bang, V. (1968b). *Epistémologie et psychologie de l'identité.* Paris: Presses Universitaires de France.
Piaget, J. (1970). Inconscient affectif et inconscient cognitif. *Raison Présente, 19,* 11–20; translated into English (1976) as: *The affective unconscious and the cognitive unconscious.* In B. Inhelder & S. Chipman (Eds.), *Piaget and his school.* New York: Springer.
Piaget, J. (1975). *L'équilibration des structures cognitives.* Paris: Presses Universitaires de France; translated into English (1977) as: *The development of thought: Equilibration of cognitive structures.* London: The Viking Press.
Piaget, J., et al. (1977). *Recherches sur l'abstraction réfléchissante* (2 volumes). Paris: Presses Universitaires de France.
Piaget, J, & Garcia, R. (1987). *Vers une logique des significations.* Murionde.
Richardson, A. (1969). *Mental imagery.* New York: Springer.
Schmid-Kitsikis, E. (1969). *L'examen des opérations de l'intelligence, Psychopathologie de l'enfant.* Neuchâtel: Delachaux et Niestlé.

Schmid-Kitsikis, E. (1976). *The cognitive mechanisms underlying problem-solving in psychotic and mentally retarded children.* In B. Inhelder and S. Chipman (Eds.), *Piaget and his school* New York: Springer.
Schmid-Kitsikis, E., & Weinstein, G. (1983). L'enfant en difficulté: une certaine conception de la formation à l'intervention psychologique. *Psychothérapies, Médecine et Hygiène, 1,* 27–35.
Schmid-Kitsikis, E. (1985a). *Théorie et clinique du fonctionnement mental.* Bruxelles: Mardaga.
Schmid-Kitsikis, E. (1985b). Some epistemological aspects of mental functioning. In V.L. Shulman, L.C.R. Resteino-Baumann & L. Butler (Eds.). *The future of Piagetian theory.* New York: Plenum Press.
Schmid-Kitsikis, E. (1985c). Clinical investigation and Piagetian experimentation. In V.L. Schulman, L.C.R. Resteino-Baumann & L. Butler (Eds.), *The future of Piagetian theory.* New York: Plenum Press.
Schmid-Kitsikis, E. (1987). Development of mental functioning: Integrative approach to psychoanalytic and psychogenetic theory. *Human Development, 30,* 189–209.
Schmid-Kitsikis, E., Bontron-Gobalet, C., Perret-Catipovic, M., Rusconi-Serpa, S., & Vionnet, S. (1987). *Explorer, symboliser, conceptualiser.* Fondation Archives Piaget.
Segal, H. (1957). Notes on symbol formation. *International Journal of Psychoanalysis.*
Segal, H. (1981). *The work of Hanna Segal. A Kleinian approach to clinical practice.* New York: Jason Aronson.
Segal, S.J. (1971). *Imagery: Current cognitive approaches.* New York: Academic Press.
Segal, S.J. (1972). Assimilation of a stimulus in the construction of an image; The Perky effect revisited. In P.W. Sheehan (Ed.), *The function and nature of imagery.* New York: Academic Press.
Sheehan, P.W. (1966). Functional similarity of imaging to perceiving: Individual differences in vividness of imagery. *Perceptual and Motor Skills, 23,* 1011–1033.
Sheehan, P.W. (1972). *The function and nature of imagery.* New York: Academic Press.
Singer, J.L. (1966). *Daydreaming.* New York: Random House.
Spitz, R. (1965). *The first year of life.* New York: International Universities Press.
Steiner, G. (1983). L'image mentale: Nouveaux aspects. *Archives de Psychologie, 51,* 355–368.
Weiner, M.L. (1975). *The cognitive unconscious. A Piagetian approach to psychotherapy.* New York: International Psychological Press.
Weiner, M.L. (1985). *Cognitive experimental therapy: An integrative ego psychotherapy.* New York: Brunner/Mazel Publishers.
Wildlocher, D. (1962). *Le Psychodrame chez l'enfant.* Paris: Presses Universitaires de France.
Winnicott, D.W. (1935). *The manic defence.* Collected papers (1958). Through paediatrics to psycho-analysis. New York: Basic Books.
Winnicott, D.W. (1971). *Playing and reality.* London: Tavistock.

Prof. Dr. Elsa Schmid-Kitsikis, F.P.S.E., Université de Genève,
24, rue Général-Dufour, CH–1211 Genève 4 (Switzerland)

Subject Index